Balance

Exercises

Balance Training Exercises for Seniors to Improve Strength

(Simple Home Exercises for Unshakeable Balance)

Andrea Celaya

Published By **Bella Frost**

Andrea Celaya

Balance Exercises: Balance Training Exercises for Seniors to Improve Strength (Simple Home Exercises for Unshakeable Balance)

ISBN   978-0-9958659-7-6

Legal & Disclaimer

The information contained in this ebook is not designed to replace or take the place of any form of medicine or professional medical advice. The information in this ebook has been provided for educational & entertainment purposes only.

The information contained in this book has been compiled from sources deemed reliable, and it is accurate to the best of the Author's knowledge; however, the Author cannot guarantee its accuracy and validity and cannot be held liable for any errors or omissions. Changes are periodically made to this book. You must consult your doctor or get professional medical advice before using any of the suggested remedies, techniques, or information in this book.

Upon using the information contained in this book, you agree to hold harmless the Author from and against any damages, costs, and expenses, including any legal fees potentially resulting from the application of any of the information provided by this guide. This disclaimer applies to any damages or injury caused by the use and application, whether directly or indirectly, of any advice or information presented, whether for breach of contract, tort, negligence, personal injury, criminal intent, or under any other cause of action.

You agree to accept all risks of using the information presented inside this book. You need to consult a professional medical practitioner in order to ensure you are both able and healthy enough to participate in this program.

Table of contents

Chapter 1: Importance Of Exercising The Body

Want to feel higher, have extra strength, and possibly add years for your lifestyles? Just exercising.

The health blessings of everyday exercising and physical hobby are difficult to deny. Everyone blessings from exercise, no matter age, sex, or bodily ability.

Need extra convincing to start moving? Check out those seven ways that exercise may result in a happier, more healthy you.

1. Exercise regulates weight

Exercise may also assist keep away from extra weight benefit or help preserve weight reduction. When you participate in physical exercise, you burn calories. The more intensive the exercising, the extra calories you burn.

Regular tours to the gym are wonderful but don't panic if you cannot discover a big block of time to training session every day. Any quantity of exercise is higher than none in any respect. To benefit the benefits of exercise, without a doubt become extra active all through your day – take the steps as opposed to the elevator or speed up your home tasks. Consistency is critical.

2. Exercise combats health problems and disorders

Worried about heart sickness? Hoping to keep away from high blood strain? No be counted what your present weight is, being energetic improves excessive-density lipoprotein (HDL) cholesterol, the "excellent" cholesterol, and it reduces harmful triglycerides. This one-two punch maintains your blood flowing smoothly, which minimizes your risk of cardiovascular issues.

Regular exercise allows save you or manipulate various fitness conditions and worries, which includes:

Stroke

Metabolic syndrome

High blood pressure

Type 2 diabetes

Depression

Anxiety

Many kinds of most cancers

Arthritis

Falls

It may additionally assist beautify cognitive function and help reduce the danger of loss of life from all causes.

three. Exercise boosts temper

Need an emotional lift? Or want to destress after a difficult day? A gymnasium exercising or brisk stroll may help. Physical exercising triggers numerous mind chemicals that may leave you feeling happier, calmer, and much less pressured. You can also experience better about your looks and your self while you workout consistently, which can also boost your confidence and beautify your vanity.

four. Exercise promotes energy

Winded through supermarket shopping or home chores? Regular bodily workout might also enhance your muscular energy and strengthen your staying power. Exercise gives oxygen and nourishment to your tissues and allows your cardiovascular gadget carry out greater efficiently. And as your heart and lung fitness enhance, you've got extra power to undertake regular obligations.

five. Exercise promotes better sleep

Struggling to snooze? Regular bodily workout may help you fall asleep quicker, experience better sleep, and deepen your sleep. Just don't exercising too near night, or you will be too stimulated to doze off.

6. Exercise brings the spark returned into your sex life

Do you experience too exhausted or too out of shape to revel in physical intimacy? Regular physical exercise can also beautify energy levels and raise your confidence on your physical appearance, which can also reinforce your intercourse existence. But there may be even more to it than that. Regular physical exercise may additionally raise arousal for women. And men who exercise constantly are much less in all likelihood to develop difficulties with erectile disorder than folks who do not exercise.

7. Exercise may be enjoyable ... and sociable!

Exercise and physical exercise may be glad. They provide you a threat to loosen up, experience the outdoors, or just indulge in matters that make you glad. Physical workout might also assist you engage with own family or buddies in an enjoyable social scenario.

So take a dancing elegance, cross trekking or be part of a football team. Find a bodily pastime you like, and simply do it. Bored? Try some thing new, or do some thing with pals or own family.

The backside line on exercising

Exercise and bodily exercise are exquisite strategies to feel higher, boom your health and feature a laugh. For most wholesome human beings, the U.S. Department of Health and Human Services recommends following exercise tips:

Aerobic hobby. Get at least a hundred and fifty minutes of moderate cardio exercising or 75 minutes of excessive cardio activity a week, or a combination of slight and strenuous hobby. The regulations advocated that you stretch out this activity over every week. To provide even extra fitness benefits and to useful resource with weight loss or maintaining weight loss, as a minimum 300 minutes per week is counseled. But even tiny quantities of bodily exercise are useful. Being active for a little quantity of time at some stage in the day may increase to carry fitness advantages.

Strength education. Do electricity training sporting events for all primary muscle organizations as a minimum two times per week. Aim to execute a single set of each exercise with a weight or resistance level hard sufficient to exhaust your muscles after around 12 to 15 repetitions.

Moderate aerobic workout consists of activities which includes brisk walking, bicycling, swimming, and mowing the garden. Vigorous aerobic exercising consists of sports which includes strolling, difficult yardwork, and cardio dance. Strength training may additionally involve using weight machines, your body weight, heavy baggage, resistance tubing or resistance paddles in the water, or interests including mountain climbing.

If you want to reduce weight, reach particular fitness targets or advantage even extra advantages, you can want to ramp up your mild cardio workout even in addition.

Chapter 2: Keeping Fit (Myth)

If you've got heard that exercise quick aerobic is the key to dropping weight or that how plenty you sweat in the course of a exercise determines how a hit it's far, it wouldn't be the first time. We talked to a personal instructor and dug up medical papers to corroborate the information so that you can stay knowledgeable. Here are some of the maximum prevalent health misconceptions, debunked.

Myth #1: 'Toning' and 'lengthening' muscular tissues

For the longest time, energy education commonly focused adult males who wanted to place on muscular bulk. Women averted it because they were counseled that in the event that they lifted big weights they might acquire "cumbersome". Instead, girls were focused with advertising and marketing phrases together with, "firming" and "lengthening" their muscle tissue. But "firming" just method gaining muscle. Hence, why your muscles seem extra "toned" as they expand and end up greater defined. To beef up your muscle tissues you need to be below a progressive overload, or in different phrases, add greater weight or greater repetitions gradually in your electricity schooling regimen.

Meanwhile, you've heard of "lengthening" your muscle mass in case you've long past to pilates, yoga, or barre elegance because the actions you're performing are intended that will help you create a "long" and "lean" appearance. "Lengthening" your muscle mass is also a piece of a stretch, considering you can't physiologically adjust the length of your muscle groups. Appearing "lean" has more to do along with your food and lower body fats than the form of interest. Although pilates, barre, and yoga classes are excellent solutions to develop your flexibility, they can't provide you "long" and "lean" muscular tissues.

Myth #2: Spot discount

Spot discount is the notion that you may burn fats from a particular phase of your frame — such as your belly — through engaging in activities for that area. You've heard this tale from some health influencers suggesting that if you do sufficient crunches, you may collect six-percent abs. When in truth, it is difficult to honestly target a unmarried location of the body to shed fats or weight. "The nice approach to lose fat in any part of your body is to devour in a calorie deficit and deal with whole body energy training," argues Onyx private teacher, Kim DiLandro.

One different issue to take into account is that fats deposited in your body, also called triglycerides, is utilized for strength. When the fats is wanted for strength it is broken down into unfastened fatty acids and glycerol. As a effect, the fats that is damaged down and utilized for fuel may originate from any portion of the body. Hence, why cannot you undertake body-particular workout routines to burn fats in that one place? Studies have additionally indicated that resistance education allows with fat discount, however the places you work out throughout the ones periods additionally don't have an effect on whether or not you lose fats in that location. "Fat discount will seem exceptional on every body and genetics plays a large impact in figuring out in which you convey it," DiLandro says.

The slogan "no ache, no benefit" is broadly used in the health quarter as a technique to motivate people to push themselves harder during their training. While it is healthful to push yourself periodically, doing it too frequently would possibly set you up for harm and set back your performance talents. In truth, constantly pushing too hard may additionally expand the overtraining syndrome, which hinders your muscle tissues' capacity to recover effectively, affects your temper, your immune device, and more. Furthermore, it might damage your capability to sleep considering that an excessive amount of hobby can overstimulate the neural machine.

Myth #3: Monthly demanding situations

Monthly difficulties appear to bombard us at the beginning of the new 12 months. They're typically within the form of a 30-day challenge that challenges you to perform a hundred squats a day or do away with dietary classes, amongst other instances. The hassle with those demanding situations is that they're simply brief-term treatments, and they might placed your health in hazard.

"Monthly meals demanding situations like detoxes or inflexible diets expand an bad connection with meals, and typically the weight loss observed is water weight that comes again instead fast after," says DiLandro. She adds that those demanding situations promise that if you could only live with one intense for a specific duration, you will miraculously see benefits, which isn't authentic. Depending on the difficulty, it might once in a while inflict extra harm than advantage.

For instance, if you have not exercised in months and all at once decide to tackle a strolling assignment, you might placed your self in hazard of damage given that most of those challenges tend to be intense and lack balance. Instead, the best approach might be to make sensible goals for yourself which can stretch beyond that month. Consult with a non-public teacher who can perform an evaluation and build a tailored program that fits your health degree and has a balanced agenda for running out and rest days.

Myth #four: Muscle confusion

Muscle

In fact, it is the weight that muscle groups adapt to. So, if you are not exercising modern overload on your exercise, then your body will maintain to adapt. Landro advocates persevering with the equal routine for weeks with an emphasis on slow overload. This includes elevating the load you are lifting, growing the variety of repetitions or sets, or converting up the velocity or period underneath stress.

Myth #5: Fasted aerobics for weight reduction

Fasted aerobic, or workout on an empty belly, has been part of the big debate in terms of weight reduction. It received prominence when bodybuilder Bill Phillips positioned it on the map in his e book, Body for Life. The concept behind practicing fasted workout is that you'll burn greater fats since your body is utilising stored fats as power as opposed to glucose.

Although you could first of all burn greater energy with the aid of acting a fasted exercise, ultimately it would not make a wonderful difference on the subject of weight reduction due to the fact what counts most is your entire every day calorie consumption. In other words, if weight loss is your aim, being in a calorie deficit is an awful lot greater critical than whether you work out fasting or now not. Studies have also shown that there has been no vast distinction in weight loss among individuals who performed fasted aerobic and people who did non-fasted aerobic.

Overall if you find you work out better on an empty belly and have a easy invoice of fitness, there's nothing incorrect with training fasting cardio. Depending on the form of workout you're appearing (including weight training), you may locate being nourished in advance is a better opportunity to preserve you from hitting a wall. If you are pregnant or have blood sugar, blood strain, or different medical difficulties, you have to contact your medical doctor before task fasted cardio or keep away from it completely.

Myth #6: Exercising to burn off food

If you comply with fitness accounts on social media, you've visible those infographics that inform you the interest same to burning off a chocolate bar or a selected form of meals. While in principle this looks as if it'd make experience, the hassle is you can't out-exercising your consuming alternatives. For one, exercising money owed for kind of 15 to 30% of your daily electricity expenditure compared on your resting metabolic price (when you're at rest), which makes use of as much as 60 to 75% of power.

Keep in thoughts every body's frame differs when it comes to how they burn calories, because it relies on things along with your weight, lean muscle groups, and interest, and studies have proven that even the time of day can also adjust what number of energy we burn. So it would be impossible to even identify how long you'll ought to exercise session to burn off a chocolate bar.

This wondering also places you at risk for disordered eating and fosters an unhealthy connection with exercising, when you consider that you'll begin connecting exercising with the simplest objective of burning off energy. Applying guilt to meals in addition supports classifying things as "good" or "horrific," some thing CNET has formerly blanketed in our listing of out of date health buzzwords.

Myth #7: Muscle may remodel into fats

This is one of the normal myths I've heard over and over again. The reality is muscle cannot develop into fats or vice versa. Fat and muscle are extraordinary tissues with one-of-a-kind cell makeups. Muscle comes in 3 paperwork: skeletal, cardiac, and easy. While frame fat (or adipose tissue) is made of triglycerides, a glycerol backbone, and 3 fatty acid chains.

"This fallacy stems from the belief that whilst you forestall running out, your body composition may additionally alternate, but the range on the size would no longer," provides DiLandro. She thinks what finally ends up taking place is you lose muscular mass thru muscle atrophy. To simplify this notion, consider while you fastidiously teach and put on muscle. Your muscular tissues develop greater obvious because you're burning more calories and hence, your fats cells cut back. Likewise, when you prevent exercise and burn fewer energy, your muscle cells decrease too. This produces the arrival that your muscle has changed into fat, whilst in fact, it's honestly your fat cells increasing.

Myth #eight: Being sore signals you had a very good exercising

Most people count on that being sore after a exercising is the finest signal that they'd a successful session. Generally, we come to be sore after we have attempted a new workout or driven ourselves more than regular. This is termed not on time onset muscle pain (DOMS), and it leaves our muscle tissues infected, and painful, and there may additionally even be stiffness and tightness. This discomfort lasts 24 to forty eight hours after your workout and typically passes on its personal, despite the fact that you could receive a rub down or foam roll to aid with restoration.

Landro thinks a higher technique to choose whether or not you had a solid workout is to research in case you're able to carry heavier or accomplish greater repetitions all through your next training session. And the greatest component is the greater you adapt to an workout, the less pain you'll get. Studies have found out this can be because of your immune gadget T-which cells resource inside the method of recuperation your muscles.

Myth #9: Eating soon after you figure out

The anabolic window of opportunity refers to the quick length after workout while you need to devour protein and carbohydrates, otherwise, you may lose out on muscle constructing — or will you? This practice has to do with new cells, tissues, and muscular tissues forming as part of your frame's reaction to exercising. Strength education breaks down muscular tissues, and when the ones muscle tissue heal and rebuild, they may be also capable of turn out to be larger and more potent. However, nutrient timing is less definitive than initially believed.

Some studies demonstrates that the belief of the anabolic window derives from the idea that exercise in a fasting country promotes muscle breakdown and keeps to achieve this put up-exercising. In this example, it'd make experience to devour a combination of protein and carbohydrates after your exercising to avoid that breakdown and rather growth muscle protein synthesis, leading to muscular development. However, in case you workout mid-day or within the nighttime after eating a meal some hours previous, it is much less required with the intention to persist with those regulations. What topics most is which you're eating your day by day requirement of protein and carbs regularly to help your muscle tissue grow and recover.

The records contained in this newsletter is for academic and informational functions most effective and isn't always supposed as fitness or clinical recommendation. Always go to a physician or other educated fitness expert approximately any inquiries you can have about a clinical situation or health dreams.

Chapter 3: How To Make Working Out Fun

Do you regularly marvel how other people can like working out? Do you regard operating out as simply one more item in your lengthy to-do list? What in case you discovered to hyperlink exercise with joy and anticipation as a substitute? If you've spent a whole lot of your existence disliking running out or equating exercising with suffering, it's time to regulate how you think and learn how to love running out.

In these days's surroundings, we're doing an increasing number of from domestic - together with working and working out. But many people find working out at home less motivating. With nobody round to guide you and encourage you to gain your fitness goals, it's less difficult to permit operating out move by the wayside. It's more critical than ever to locate a way to make running out gratifying.

Is it feasible to go from disliking running out to without a doubt loving it? The answer is sure - if you are decided to regulate your angle and make the changes required.

Like learning any new capability, knowing how to love exercise is a part mentality and element practice. By adopting the mentality that workout is glad, you're able to embrace health as a part of a comprehensive fitness plan. Learning the way to appreciate operating out becomes a exquisite device for improving your fitness and achieving the physique you preference – and the terrific life you deserve.

Aerobic workout for weight loss is a laugh, and there are numerous strategies to parent out a way to love running out.

What are the core standards in the back of gaining knowledge of how to appreciate running out? The U.S. Office of Disease Prevention and Health Promotion claims that there are five critical components in appreciating exercising and making it a dependancy: pleasure, self-efficacy, social assist, accountability and integration into your everyday life. Since the maximum successful fitness routine is one you'll stick with, the first element – studying a way to love exercise – is critical.

Building self-self belief is also vital. If you're afraid or uncertain, your anxieties will damage your tries to exercising. Social assist plays a full-size element in the way to revel in operating out, as human beings are social beings suffering from their peer companies. Those peer businesses sell duty, every other vital element in gaining knowledge of a way to love operating out. And by using incorporating exercise into your normal routine, it will become a habit. From here, you're capable of exercise session in your fitness and amusing.

TIPS FOR HOW TO ENJOY EXERCISE

Exercise, whether to drop extra pounds or enhance your health, may be fun. There are methods to parent out a way to begin loving working out instead of hating it.

1. CHANGE YOUR BELIEFS ABOUT WORKING OUT

Want to learn how to love exercise? It all begins with assessing your thoughts and replacing negative ideals with superb ones. Many of your perspectives have been hooked up in childhood. If you participated in uninteresting P.E. Lessons or have been pressured to be at the track team whilst you disliked jogging, you in all likelihood developed the notion that running out became some thing to be endured instead of loved.

Take time to discover your thoughts around workout: Which are negative and which might be fantastic? Where did the horrific ideals originate from? Are they still valid for your grownup lifestyles or are you clinging to outdated notions that no longer help you? Once you apprehend which ideas are proscribing you from getting to know the way to experience running out, you may consciousness on changing them into the high-quality thoughts that assist you attain your targets.

2. ADJUST YOUR FOCUS

Many people have issues mastering a way to revel in running out because they are focused on simply one outcome: weight reduction.

When you keep in mind workout merely as a method to govern weight, it becomes a "need to" or an responsibility. As Tony advises, don't "have to" throughout your self! Instead of considering operating workout as a way to shed pounds, remind yourself that your frame is yours to attend to and that each unmarried desire you are making – whether exact or dangerous – has the strength to advantage or injure you.

When you begin targeting revitalizing your body, improving your health and enriching your lifestyles, you will start to understand exercise as a wholesome choice as opposed to an duty. Then running exercise will become a herbal extension of looking after oneself.

This alteration in your mentality may additionally assist you learn how to experience running out at domestic. You will not need the social strain element to urge you to workout. When you're exercise for your self and now not for others, it is lots less difficult to feel motivated.

three. FIND THE RIGHT TYPE OF WORKOUT

How to like exercising is all about choosing the correct type of interest. Take a while and replicate back to a length while you liked physical activities. Were you with friends, in a crew or going solo? In a lovely outdoor surroundings? Participating in a game? Working out does no longer have to entail going to a health club and strolling on a treadmill for half an hour. It may truely entail participating in bodily sports you experience.

Taking a karate elegance or rehearsing your child's cheerleading recurring with them offers the same fitness blessings as running or using the elliptical system. Many individuals bypass workout due to the fact they expect it has to appear a selected way to qualify as "operating out." This honestly isn't proper. Any sort of physical interest that enhances your coronary heart fee is a shape of exercising. When you discover an hobby that makes you blissful, you'll stay up for it in place of heading off it. This is one of the finest matters you can do while you're learning a way to make working out pleasing.

4. MAKE SURE YOU HAVE THE ENERGY TO EXERCISE

Learning the way to love working out is a alternatively intimidating venture whilst you barely have sufficient power to do your simple every day responsibilities. Joint soreness and pain may additionally use up your enthusiasm and depart you asking a way to make working out great.

If a lack of power or irritation are stopping you from operating out, you want to study your wellknown life-style. Are you consuming clean whole meals and rich in fiber? Are you ingesting plenty of water and taking the correct supplements? Do you've got effective strategies to address strain?

Poor food, loss of self-care and a build-up of strain may additionally sap your vitality. Working from domestic paired with extra child care duties might depart you feeling fatigued and frustrated. How to love working out lowers pretty low for your listing of priorities while it's all you could do to truely get through the day. After a day of working from home, it's not very inspirational to merely step into the subsequent room for your workout.

If your life-style is a barrier to knowledge the way to admire workout, accept Tony Robbins' 10-Day Challenge. You'll deliver your self the gift of extra energy, a healthful food regimen, most effective interest and physical health. Once you are making healthful changes, you'll free up the energy required to find out the way to love operating out.

five. CREATE TIME TO WORK OUT

You can't discover ways to experience exercise if you don't create the time for your agenda to exercise session. If you move into your work out feeling rushed or that you are sacrificing too much of it slow by using running out, you aren't going to enjoy your revel in.

Maybe you generally squeezed your exercise in in your manner domestic from the workplace, and with remote work, your agenda has gone wild. Or perhaps you've reached that iciness fitness rut, when it receives dark early and all you need to do after work is go home.

Or perhaps you accept as true with that in case you don't have time to exercising within the morning, you might as nicely now not hassle - however this isn't real. While morning sporting activities are an exhilarating way to set a exquisite tone in your day, it isn't the simplest time you can squeeze an effective exercising in. Working exercise at any hour of the day is higher than no longer working out in any respect. Oftentimes, the notion which you don't have time to exercising is handiest an excuse that arises out of your limiting ideals as opposed to a proper scheduling constraint.

The reality is, you have to make time to do the belongings you enjoy — and that includes operating out. Don't create excuses - rather, find a solution. Set up your elliptical in front of your TV and work out as you watch your favored comedy. Take 15-minute breaks at work and stroll around the block. While your teen is at soccer practice, strength-stroll round the sphere. When you recognize you don't need to cut out crucial elements of your lifestyles to work out, you can discover ways to experience operating out without feeling responsible.

6. CREATE AN INSPIRING SPACE

Want to discover the way to enjoy operating out at domestic? Your environment can also have more to do with it than you believe. While many of us don't have room for an entire yoga studio in our residing areas, placing off a portion of a room or utilising a room divider may work just as well. A basement is another first rate preference for maintaining a few gadgets of home gym gadget. You don't need a ton of room. Just enough to make your exercise excellent.

Music is another vital aspect of mastering a way to love workout. In one study, researchers tested 3 groups of individuals: people who listened to music whilst exercise, those who listened to a podcast and those who listened to not anything.

Music improved satisfaction by means of 28% in comparison to people with no auditory stimulation and by 13% as compared to folks who listened to a podcast. Researchers observed that given that music evoked a greater high-quality emotional kingdom during workout, music is a splendid device for learning the way to revel in operating out – and you could utilize it whether or not your training area is in your private home or within the large outside.

7. LEARN TO BE MORE ADAPTABLE

Humans searching for predictability, even in our workout regimens. We're additionally especially sociable people, difficult-stressed to paintings together and revel in gatherings. When it comes to mastering how to make operating out satisfying, there may be strength in numbers. One research indicated that our social networks impact our exercise-associated behavior. Participants who frolicked with healthy companions were more likely to efficiently reduce weight and enjoy workout than the ones whose peers were now not oriented towards healthier dwelling.

If you're having problems getting to know a way to experience operating out at home without your social community, pass your interest to construct a growth mindset so one can inspire you to grasp new things.

In addition to adjusting your thinking, mix up your routine, too. Variety is also one in all our middle human desires, so regulate up your fitness program every week to avoid turning into bored. Join a virtual fitness venture or a web community in which you can achieve encouragement. Connecting with other individuals in similar instances is a first-rate approach to don't forget a way to recognize working out. Remember what Tony says: "Every challenge is a present — with out problems we would no longer develop." How can you utilize your present limitations to gain progress in your lifestyles?

Chapter 4: How To Get Started (60+)

Do you often surprise how different people can like working out? Do you regard operating out as simply one extra object for your prolonged to-do list? What in case you discovered to hyperlink exercise with joy and anticipation rather? If you've spent an awful lot of your lifestyles disliking running out or equating exercising with struggling, it's time to adjust how you observed and discover ways to love running out.

In today's environment, we're doing an increasing number of from domestic - such as operating and running out. But many individuals discover working out at homeless motivating. With nobody around to aid you and inspire you to attain your fitness goals, it's less difficult to allow working out move by the wayside. It's extra vital than ever to locate how to make running out pleasing.

Is it possible to move from disliking operating out to definitely loving it? The solution is yes - in case you are determined to modify your perspective and make the adjustments required.

Like mastering any new capability, knowing how to love exercising is part mentality and part practice. By adopting the mentality that workout is happy, you're able to embrace health as a part of a comprehensive fitness plan. Learning the way to appreciate working out turns into a notable device for improving your health and accomplishing the physique you choice – and the awesome life you deserve.

Aerobic workout for weight reduction is amusing, and there are various techniques to figure out the way to love operating out.

What are the middle ideas at the back of getting to know a way to respect working out? The U.S. Office of Disease Prevention and Health Promotion claims that there are five important additives in appreciating workout and making it a habit: pride, self-efficacy, social aid, accountability, and integration into your regular life. Since the most successful health routine is one you'll keep on with, the primary issue – gaining knowledge of a way to love workout – is important.

Building self-self belief is likewise crucial. If you're afraid or uncertain, your anxieties will harm your attempts to exercise. Social aid performs a good sized part in the way to enjoy working out, as humans are social beings tormented by their peer companies. Those peer corporations promote responsibility, any other crucial factor of studying the way to love working out. And by incorporating exercise into your everyday habitual, it turns into a habit. From right here, you're capable of work out in your health and a laugh.

TIPS FOR HOW TO ENJOY EXERCISE

Exercise, whether to shed extra pounds or enhance your fitness, may be a laugh. There are techniques to discern out a way to start loving working out instead of hating it.

1. CHANGE YOUR BELIEFS ABOUT WORKING OUT

Want to discover ways to love exercising? It all starts offevolved with assessing your mind and replacing terrible beliefs with wonderful ones. Many of your views had been established in adolescence. If you participated in tedious P.E. Guides or had been forced to be on the song team whilst you loathed strolling, you probable formed the mind-set that working out changed into some thing to be endured as a substitute than loved.

Take time to discover your mind around workout: Which are terrible and which are high-quality? Where did the awful ideals originate from? Are they still legitimate on your person existence or are you clinging to outmoded notions that now not assist you? Once you recognize which thoughts are limiting you from getting to know how to revel in running out, you can consciousness on converting them into positive thoughts that help you attain your targets.

2. ADJUST YOUR FOCUS

Many people have troubles studying the way to enjoy working out due to the fact they may be concentrated on simply one final results: weight reduction.

When you remember exercise simply as a technique to govern weight, it turns into a "ought to" or an duty. As Tony advises, don't "need to" all over your self! Instead of considering running workout as a technique to shed pounds, remind your self that your body is yours to attend to and that each unmarried preference you're making — whether or not desirable or dangerous — has the energy to gain or injure you.

When you begin targeting revitalizing your frame, enhancing your fitness, and enriching your existence, you'll begin to perceive exercise as a wholesome option as opposed to an responsibility. Then running exercising will become a herbal extension of taking care of oneself. This alteration to your mentality can also help you learn how to experience working out at domestic. You will now not need the social stress factor to induce you to training session. When you're exercising for your self and now not for others, it's a lot simpler to experience influenced.

three. FIND THE RIGHT TYPE OF WORKOUT

How to love workout is all about deciding on the precise form of hobby. Take some time and replicate on a length while you appreciated bodily activities. Were you with friends, in a group, or going solo? In a lovely outdoor surroundings? Participating in a game? Working out does now not need to entail going to a health club and walking on a treadmill for 1/2 an hour. It may simply entail participating in bodily sports you experience.

Taking a karate elegance or rehearsing your toddler's cheerleading habitual with them gives the identical fitness blessings as jogging or using the elliptical system. Many people bypass workout because they assume it has to appear in a selected way to qualify as "operating out." This truly isn't proper. Any kind of physical hobby that boosts your heart price is a form of workout. When you find out an pastime that makes you glad, you'll look ahead to it rather than heading off it. This is one of the finest matters you can do even as you're learning the way to make operating out satisfying.

4. MAKE SURE YOU HAVE THE ENERGY TO EXERCISE

Learning how to love operating out is a as an alternative intimidating challenge while you barely have sufficient power to do your primary daily obligations. Joint discomfort and soreness may also deplete your enthusiasm and leave you asking a way to make working out nice.

If a loss of power or irritation is stopping you from working out, you need to check your preferred lifestyle. Are you eating clean complete meals rich in fiber? Are you consuming lots of water and taking the appropriate supplements? Do you've got effective techniques to deal with stress?

Poor meals, lack of self-care, and a build-up of pressure may additionally sap your energy. Working from domestic paired with extra childcare duties may depart you feeling fatigued and pissed off. How to love operating out lowers quite low for your listing of priorities whilst it's all you may do to actually get through the day. After a day of working from domestic, it's not very inspirational to simply step into the subsequent room for your exercise.

If your lifestyle is a barrier to knowledge how to respect the exercising, be given Tony Robbins' 10-Day Challenge. You'll deliver your self the present of extra strength, a healthy food regimen, premier attention, and bodily fitness. Once you're making healthy modifications, you'll loose up the power required to discover the way to love running out.

five. CREATE TIME TO WORK OUT

You can't learn how to recognize exercise if you don't make the time for your schedule to workout. If you stroll into your workout feeling hurried or which you are sacrificing too much of some time by means of working out, you aren't going to experience your enjoy.

Maybe you normally squeezed your exercise in for your manner domestic from the office, and with far flung paintings, your agenda has gone wild. Or perhaps you've reached that wintry weather fitness rut while it receives dark early and all you want to do after paintings is pass home.

Or perhaps you believe that if you don't have time to exercise within the morning, you might as nicely not bother - but this isn't real. While morning sporting events are a thrilling manner to set a first-rate tone for your day, it isn't the best time you could squeeze an effective workout in. Working out at any hour of the day is higher than now not working out at all. Oftentimes, the thought that you don't have time to exercise is best an excuse that arises from your restricting beliefs instead of a genuine scheduling constraint.

The truth is, you need to make time to do the things you revel in — and that includes running out. Don't create excuses - rather, discover a answer. Set up your elliptical in the front of your TV and exercise session as you watch your favored comedy. Take 15-minute breaks at work and walk around the block. While your teenager is at football practice, strength-walk around the sphere. When you apprehend you don't need to cut out vital elements of your lifestyles to workout, you can discover ways to experience operating out without feeling responsible.

6. CREATE AN INSPIRING SPACE

Want to discover a way to enjoy running out at home? Your environment can also have extra to do with it than you believe. While lots of us don't have room for a whole yoga studio in our dwelling spaces, placing off a portion of a room or utilizing a room divider may fit just as properly. A basement is another exceptional choice for keeping some items of domestic health club device. You don't need a ton of room. Just enough to make your workout high-quality.

Music is another vital thing of mastering how to love exercising. In one observe, researchers tested three groups of individuals: individuals who listened to track at the same time as exercise, folks that listened to a podcast, and those who listened to not anything.

Music improved pride by way of 28% compared to those with no auditory stimulation and by means of thirteen% as compared to those who listened to a podcast. Researchers located that on account that track evoked a more first-class emotional nation all through exercise, tune is a amazing device for learning how to enjoy working out – and you can put it to use whether your schooling area is in your home or the vast exterior.

7. LEARN TO BE MORE ADAPTABLE

Humans are trying to find predictability, even in our exercising regimens. We're also especially sociable humans, difficult-wired to work collectively and enjoy gatherings. When it involves gaining knowledge of the way to make running out satisfying, there may be power in numbers. One research indicated that our social networks impact our exercise-associated conduct. Participants who frolicked with wholesome companions had been much more likely to efficaciously reduce weight and revel in workout than those whose friends had been now not orientated toward healthier living.

If you're having issues mastering how to enjoy working out at domestic without your social network, circulate your interest to constructing a boom mind-set in order to encourage you to grasp new things.

In addition to adjusting your questioning, mix up your ordinary, too. Variety is likewise certainly one of our middle human wishes, so adjust your health application each week to keep away from becoming bored. Join a digital fitness task or a web community in which you may achieve encouragement. Connecting with other people in similar instances is a outstanding method to recalling how to appreciate running out. Remember what Tony says: "Every challenge is a gift — with out problems, we'd not grow." How can you utilize your gift limitations to acquire development in your life?

Chapter 5: How To Start Exercising And Stick To It

Overcoming difficulties in workout

If you're having issues organising an exercise regimen or following through, you're now not on my own. Many folks have issue getting out of the sedentary rut, despite our exceptional efforts.

You already understand there are many wonderful advantages to exercise—from boosting strength, mood, sleep, and fitness to lowering worry, pressure, and depression. And thorough exercising instructions and schooling routines are most effective a click away. But if know-how how and why to workout become sufficient, we'd all be in form. Making exercise a addiction calls for extra—you need the best mentality and a smart technique.

While realistic issues like a busy schedule or horrific health may make exercise difficult, for maximum of us, the primary impediments are mental. Maybe it's a loss of self-self belief that hinders you from taking desirable movements, or your drive rapidly flares out, or you turn out to be easily disheartened and end. We've all been there for some time.

Whatever your age or health degree—even in case you've in no way exercised an afternoon for your life —there are measures you may take to make workout much less daunting and unsightly and more blissful and herbal.

Ditch the all-or-not anything approach. You do not need to spend hours in a health club or push yourself into repetitive or unpleasant activities you dislike to experience the physical and intellectual advantages of exercising. A little exercise is higher than not anything. Adding without a doubt mild quantities of bodily exercising in your weekly habitual can also have a extraordinary have an effect on to your mental and emotional fitness.

Be mild to yourself. Research shows that self-compassion complements the possibility that you may succeed in any given try. So, do not beat your self up over your physique, your present health degree, or your alleged lack of willpower. All a good way to do is demotivate you. Instead, have a look at your previous mistakes and dangerous choices as chances to research and improve.

Check your expectancies. You failed to fall out of form overnight, and you are not going to speedy alter your physique both. Expecting an excessive amount of, too soon handiest leads to dissatisfaction. Try not to get discouraged by using what you can't do or how far you need to visit obtain your health objectives. Instead of stressing outcomes, focus on consistency. While the blessings in mood and electricity levels may additionally arrive swiftly, the bodily payback will come in time.

Excuses for now not exercising

Making excuses for now not exercise? Whether it's lack of time or electricity or dread of the gym, there are solutions.

Busting the top workout excuses

Excuse 1: "I loathe exercise."

Solution: Many people sense the identical. If sweating at a fitness center or pounding a treadmill isn't your idea of a wonderful time, try and find an activity which you do revel in—including dancing—or couple bodily workout with some thing extra amusing. Take a walk at lunchtime in a picturesque park, for instance, stroll laps of an air-conditioned mall even as window shopping, walk, run, cycle with a pal, or pay attention on your favourite tune as you circulate.

Excuse 2: "I'm too busy."

Solution: Even the busiest among us may additionally locate spare time in our day for significant things. It's your choice to make health a concern. And don't expect you need an entire hour for a strong exercise. Short five-, 10-, or 15-minute bursts of motion can be quite powerful—so, too, can % all of your exercising right into a handful of sessions over the weekend. If you're too busy at some stage in the week, arise and begin exercise over the weekend when you have extra time.

Excuse three: "I'm too tired."

Solution: It may additionally seem contradictory, but physical workout is a effective choose-me-up that lowers exhaustion and increases electricity degrees in the long time. With normal exercising, you'll feel considerably greater invigorated, refreshed, and aware at all times.

Excuse four: "I'm too fats," "I'm too vintage," or "My fitness isn't exact enough."

Solution: It's in no way too past due to start growing your electricity and bodily health, even whether or not you're a senior or a confessed couch potato who has never exercised earlier than. Very few fitness or weight concerns take workout out of the query, so talk to your medical doctor about a secure routine.

Excuse 5: "Exercise is simply too tough and painful."

Solution: "No ache, no gain" is an antiquated way of thinking about exercise. Exercise shouldn't harm. And you don't have to push yourself till you're bathed in sweat or every muscle hurts to acquire results. You may additionally expand your power and fitness by means of on foot, swimming, or even playing golfing, gardening, or cleansing the house.

Excuse 6: "I'm not athletic."

Solution: Still suffer nightmares from PE? You don't must be athletic or extremely-coordinated to come to be healthy. Focus on easy methods to elevate your interest level, along with taking walks, swimming, or sincerely doing greater around the home. Anything that gets you shifting will paintings.

How an awful lot exercise do you want?

The principal factor to don't forget whilst starting an workout routine is that something is constantly better than not anything. Going for a touch walk is most excellent to lounging on the couch; one minute of motion will assist you lose more weight than no activity in any respect. That said, the contemporary tenet for most individuals is to gain as a minimum one hundred fifty minutes of moderate exercise each week. You'll get there via workout for half-hour, five days every week. Can't locate half-hour for your nerve-racking schedule? It's perfect to interrupt matters up. Two 15-minute physical games or three 10-minute workout routines might be just as useful.

How hard do I need to exercising?

Whether an hobby is a low, moderate, or vigorous intensity varies in step with your health degree. As a widespread guideline, though:

Low-depth interest: You can without difficulty chat in entire sentences, and even sing.

Moderate depth: You can talk in full sentences, however no longer sing.

Vigorous intensity: You are too breathless to talk in whole terms.

For most people, striving for moderate-intensity exercise is adequate to beautify their overall health. You should breathe a bit heavier than common, however not be out of breath. Your frame ought to sense hotter as you walk, but not overheat or sweat excessively. While anybody is one-of-a-kind, don't expect that making ready for a marathon is better than training for a 5K or 10K. There's no want to overdo it.

For extra at the forms of workout, you need to include and the way hard you must training session, see Best Exercises for Health and Weight Loss.

Getting started securely

If you have by no means exercised earlier than, or it's been a large duration of time due to the fact that you've undertaken any extreme physical pastime, hold the following health concerns in thoughts:

Health problems? Get clinical clearance ahead. If you have got health troubles which include confined mobility, coronary heart ailment, bronchial asthma, diabetes, or excessive blood pressure, discuss them along with your medical doctor earlier than you begin to workout.

Warm-up. Warm up with dynamic stretches—active moves that heat and flex the muscle groups you'll be the use of, together with leg kicks, walking lunges, or arm swings—and by way of executing a slower, less difficult version of the next exercising. For instance, in case you're going to run, heat up by means of strolling. Or if you're doing weights, start with some modest repetitions.

Cool down. After your exercising, it is vital to take a couple of minutes to cool down and allow your coronary heart fee to go back to its resting charge. A short jog or walk after a run, for instance, or some slight stretches after strength education may additionally help lessen soreness and harm.

Drink lots of water. Your frame features pleasant while it is properly-hydrated. Failing to drink sufficient water even as you are exerting your self over a longer period, specially in hot climate, can be deadly.

Listen in your frame. If you revel in ache or soreness whilst going out, prevent! If you feel better after a little pause, you can slowly and punctiliously maintain your exercise. But don't try to force thru struggling. That's a guaranteed method for harm.

How to make workout a habit that remains

There is a motive such a lot of New Year's plans crash and burn before February receives round. And it is now not which you simply do not have what it takes. Science informs us that there's a accurate method to growing conduct that bear. Follow those measures to make health considered one of them.

Start small and gain momentum

A purpose of exercising for half-hour a day, five days a week may additionally seem extremely good. But how likely are you to comply with thru? The greater ambitious your intention, the much more likely you're to fail, sense terrible approximately it, and end. It's ideal to begin with easy fitness targets you know you could achieve. As you meet them, you'll collect self-confidence and momentum. Then you could pass directly to more disturbing objectives.

Make it automated using triggers

Triggers are one of the keys to achievement in terms of building an exercise addiction. Research reveals that the most chronic exercisers depend upon them. Triggers are simply reminders—a time of day, area, or cue—that start an involuntary reaction. They set your habitual on autopilot, so there is nothing to reflect onconsideration on or determine on. The alarm clock goes off and you are out the door on your stroll. You leave paintings for the day and pass without delay to the gymnasium. You undercover agent your shoes proper beside the bed and you're up and going. Find strategies to weave them into your day to make exercise a no-brainer.

Reward your self

People who workout often tend to achieve this because of the rewards it brings to their lives, which include more strength, better sleep, and a extra sense of nicely-being. However, these have a tendency to be lengthy-time period rewards. When you're starting an workout software, it is vital to provide your self on the spot rewards whilst you entire a workout or attain a brand new fitness aim. Choose something you stay up for, but do not permit your self to do until after exercise. It may be something as easy as having a warm bath or a favourite cup of espresso.

Choose sports that make you feel happy and assured

If your workout is unpleasant or makes you feel clumsy or inept, you are not going to stay with it. Don't pick out activities like jogging or lifting weights on the gymnasium simply due to the fact you consider that is what you should do. Instead, choose activities that suit your way of life, potential, and taste.

Set yourself up for success

Schedule it. You don't attend meetings and appointments spontaneously, you time table them. If you are having hassle fitting exercise into your schedule, do not forget it an essential appointment with yourself and mark it in your every day schedule.

Make it smooth on yourself. Plan your exercises throughout the time of day whilst you're most wide awake and lively. If you are now not a morning individual, for example, don't undermine your self with the aid of planning to exercising earlier than paintings.

Remove limitations. Plan in advance for anything that might get within the way of workout. Do you generally tend to expire of time within the morning? Get your exercising clothes out the night time before so you're ready to move as soon as you arise. Do you bypass your night exercise in case you pass domestic first? Keep a workout bag inside the car, so that you can go out directly from work.

Hold your self accountable. Commit to another person. If you have a exercise friend ready, you're less willing to miss out. Or ask a chum or family member to check in in your development. Announcing your objectives in your social circle (either online or in individual) may help keep you on course.

Tips for making workout more gratifying

As formerly indicated, you are notably much more likely to stick to an exercising habitual it is exciting and enjoyable. No amount of strength of mind is going to preserve you going long-time period with an exercise you despise.

Think beyond the fitness center

Does the notion of going to the fitness center fill you with dread? If you find the gym inconvenient, expensive, intimidating, or honestly uninteresting, it really is ok. There are many exercising options to weight rooms and aerobic device.

For many, definitely getting outside makes all of the difference. You may also enjoy walking outside, in which you can revel in alone time and nature, even in case you hate treadmills.

Just approximately each person can discover a physical activity they enjoy. But you can need to assume past the standard strolling, swimming, and biking options. Here are a few activities you may discover fun:

Chapter 6: Best Warming Up Exercise

The Benefits Of Warming Up Pre-Workout

"Warming up before your cardio or power training consultation is vital for heading off harm," explains Janeil Mason, a head teacher at Brrrn in New York, who also holds an MS in exercising physiology. "A respectable heat-up also prepares your fearful system and muscle groups to feature satisfactory for the duration of your exercising."

Moving through a few pre-exercise stretches might even provide your mind a lift. "It's going to help to prepare now not just the muscular tissues and joints into that posture," says Dr. Jen Fraboni, a physical therapist. "however it is also going to help in conditioning the mind to grasp what movement styles they're going into." Talk approximately a win-win.

How To Warm Up Properly

Just touching your ft might not accomplish the job. Fraboni advocates dynamic stretches, or movement stretches, to get your muscle groups geared up for top overall performance. "We understand that from research, easy static stretching might also from time to time block muscle feature," she explains. "We don't need to hinder what we're going to do—we want to make the frame extra enthusiastic, extra inflamed."

She additionally believes it's an excellent concept to recognize your boundaries and to reflect onconsideration on your unique variety of motion when you heat up. You do not need to overdo it with the aid of forcing your frame right into a role it is not geared up for (pain!). "Moving into calm, managed, lively periods is prime," Fraboni provides.

Convinced? Choose 4 to 5 of Mason's actions beneath, then perform every for 30 to 60 seconds. They work excellently no matter what form of hobby is at the application, from leaping rope to Pilates. Just give attention to the techniques on the way to first-class in shape your exercise (lower body, upper body, and many others.), Fraboni advises. Now, who's equipped to warmth things?

1

Arm Reach

How to: Begin in a status stance, along with your ft wider than hip-width aside. Pivot for your proper foot and swing your right arm over your chest. Twist your torso and upper frame in the same manner. Immediately repeat with the alternative arm. Continue for 30 to 60 seconds.

2

Side Reach

How to: Begin in a status stance, together with your toes wider than hip-width apart. Lean your frame to the right side, bending your proper knee barely. At the equal time, expand your left arm to the sky at a diagonal, in alignment with the relaxation of your frame. Stretch your left leg lengthy.

Immediately repeat on the opposite aspect. Continue for 30 to 60 seconds.

3

Hip Rotations

How to: Start in a status stance, with ft wider than hip-width aside. Bend your palms, and placed your hands behind your head. Bend your knee as you increase one leg. Circle that leg over your frame, up toward your chest, then backtrack to the beginning role. Repeat on the alternative facet. Continue for 30 to 60 seconds.

four

Knees Lift

How to: Start in a standing stance, with ft wider than hip-width aside. Bend your fingers, setting your hands at the back of your head. Lift one leg closer to your body, bending your knee as you do, as if you were attempting to touch your rib cage along with your knee. Continue for 30 to 60 seconds.

five

Lateral Lunge With Balance

How to: Stand together with your ft hip-width aside, hands at your side. Take a robust stride to the right, then push your hips lower back, bending your right knee and reducing your body till your proper knee is bent 90 ranges. Push returned to an upright posture, at the same time as you elevate your knee and draw it into your chest along with your hands. Continue for 30 to 60 seconds on the right side, then pass to the left.

6

Lateral Lunge With Reach

How to: Stand along with your ft wider than shoulder-width aside, arms at your side. With your proper hand, reach down in the direction of your foot, reducing your frame until your left knee is bent ninety ranges. Immediately repeat on the other side. Continue for 30 to 60 seconds.

7

Squat To Raised Heel

How to: Stand with your heels wider than shoulder-distance apart, then flip your toes open slightly. Bend your knees, attain your hips back, and sink into a squat. Drop your fingers down among your legs. Then, press into your heels to get up, while you loop your palms out to the side. At the height, pull your hands instantly up and rise onto your ft. Continue for 30 to 60 seconds.

eight

Squat With Reach

How to: Stand together with your heels wider than shoulder-distance aside, then flip your feet open slightly. Bend your knees, attain your hips returned, and sink right into a squat. Drop your fingers down between your legs. Then, press into your heels to get up, while you raise your arms straight overhead. Continue for 30 to 60 seconds.

nine

Plank Walk Out

How to: Start in a status posture. Bend down until your fingers contact the ground. Slowly circulate your arms ahead until you get into a plank posture. Pause for a 2d, then walk your palms returned towards your toes. Return to status. Continue for 30 to 60 seconds.

10

Jumping Jack

How to: Stand together with your toes hip distance apart, and your palms at your facets. Then, simultaneously extend your palms out to the sides and above your head, and hop your feet out so they are little greater than shoulder-width apart. Without hesitating, swiftly reverse the motion. Repeat for 30 to 60 seconds.

Chapter 7: Workout Routine (15 Minutes)

If you need to get in a robust exercising however you've most effective got 15 mins to spare, we have a splendid alternative for you.

The 15-minute total-body exercise underneath, devised via Juan Hidalgo, Los Angeles–primarily based licensed private trainer and institution health teacher, doesn't want a single piece of device to accomplish.

So you truely can virtually prevent whatever you're doing and rapid hammer out a workout (in case you so preference)—ideal for those people who need to get in a few shape of interest on a hectic day but can't always go to the health club.

This rapid total-body workout is brief yet tough, so you'll sense like to procure in a full-duration consultation in a fragment of the time.

And it leaves no major muscle group unaffected.

"It's intended to goal the overall body, rotating between decrease body, higher frame, plyometrics, and middle education," Hidalgo provides, this means that you'll mark both aerobic and energy physical activities off your list in simplest 15 mins.

The first-class part?

You don't need a unmarried piece of equipment.

You'll be pushing, pulling, squatting, and helping your frame weight.

Trust us, you're going to experience it.

If you want to make this exercising even extra of a aerobic mission, Hidalgo advises limiting relaxation time between sets.

You may additionally even opt to omit relaxation absolutely in case you want to keep your coronary heart charge excessive for the duration of and without a doubt paintings up a sweat.

You may even make the exercise greater strenuous by way of making it longer—clearly add every other set or two, Hidalgo adds. If you're new to those workouts and nonetheless looking for out what intensity works for you, start with the units and rest intervals Hidalgo advises underneath.

As you develop acquainted with the exercises, you can vary it as much as personalize it to you and your fitness degree.

1

Jumping

Jack

Start standing erect along with your fingers by means of your facets.

Jump both legs out while lifting each arms over your head till your hands' contact.

Return to the beginning function.

Continue this exercising for 1 minute.

squat to alternating curtsy lunge

2

Squat to Curtsy Lunge

Stand along with your ft slightly wider than hip-width apart, feet slightly grew to become out, and palms at your aspects or in front of your chest (as indicated) (as shown).

Engage your center and hold your chest up and again flat as you transfer your weight into your heels, push your hips returned, and bend your knees to drop right into a squat.

Drive through your heels to face and clench your glutes on the top.

Then, step your right foot diagonally behind you and drop your right knee until it almost touches the floor.

Your front knee must bend to more or less 90 degrees.

Drive through your left heel to face lower back up and go back to the beginning posture.

Continue this interest, swapping sides for the curtsy lunge every time, for 1 minute.

three

High Knees

Stand with your ft hip-width apart.

Run in region, pushing your knees up closer to your chest as excessive as possible.

You may both maintain your hands in front of you to satisfy your knees or pump them at the side of your legs.

Keep your chest raised, and middle engaged, and land lightly on the balls of your toes.

Continue for 1 minute.

pushup to shoulder faucet

4

Push-up to Shoulder Tap

Start in a excessive plank, shoulders squarely over your wrists, arms shoulder-width apart, hands flat, legs stretched at the back of you, middle and glutes engaged.

Bend your elbows and drop your body to the ground.

Drop for your knees if required (preserve your core engaged even in the modified posture) (preserve your center engaged even in the modified role).

Push through the fingers of your hands to straighten your hands.

Now contact your proper hand in your left shoulder, and then your left hand for your right shoulder.

Engage your core and glutes to preserve your hips as constant as feasible in order that they're now not swinging backward and forward.

To make this less difficult, recall parting your legs a bit greater.

Continue, alternating between a push-up and two shoulder taps, for 1 minute.

five

Plyo Lunge

Stand along with your feet collectively.

Step returned about 2 ft along with your left foot, landing at the ball of your left foot and maintaining your heel off the ground.

Bend both knees until your right quad and left shin are parallel to the floor, your frame tilting slightly ahead in order that your again is flat.

Your proper knee should be over your proper foot, and your butt and core ought to be engaged.

Push via both feet to jump directly up, swinging your palms above to generate speed.

In the air, switch legs, so that your proper foot is now behind you and your left is in the front.

As you land, drop into a lunge before instantly jumping once more.

Continue this motion, switching legs, for 1 minute.

6

Sit up Glute Bridge

Start laying in your lower back with your fingers at your aspects, knees bent, and toes flat on the ground hip-width apart.

Using your abs, roll your frame up until you're sitting upright.

You may additionally both go your palms in front of your chest or preserve them instantly out by means of your aspects.

Slowly drop backtrack to the starting function.

Squeeze your glutes and abs and push via your heels to raise your hips some inches off the floor till your frame bureaucracy a instantly line from your shoulders in your knees.

Pause and clench your glutes at the peak, then gently descend your hips to go back to the beginning function.

Continue this activity, alternating between sit-u.S.A.And glute bridges, for 1 minute.

7

Finisher: Broad Jump to Burpee

Stand with your toes shoulder-width aside and fingers by way of your sides.

Bend your knees right into a squat and bounce forward about a foot, touchdown in a squat.

Reach forward to put your palms at the ground, shoulder-width apart.

Kick your legs instantly out at the back of you right into a excessive plank together with your arms piled at the back of your shoulders.

Bend your elbows to drop your chest to the ground.

Push your body lower back up to a high plank and hop your feet closer to your arms so your lower frame is in a squat.

Backpedal to the beginning role.

Continue this exercise for 1 minute.

Chapter 8: Muscle Recovery

While muscle aches are every now and then simply part of difficult your body and getting more potent, there are things you could do to help. Use those hints to hurry up your muscle healing so that you can maintain running toward your fitness and health goals!

How to speed up muscle restoration

The Sweat Trainers regularly receive questions from the Community about how to relieve sore muscular tissues after a exercise. Here are some proven suggestions to ease those aches and assist you get returned in your education sooner:

Hydrate

Drinking water is important in your standard health and publish-exercising recovery, such as muscle repair. It's properly to intention for approximately two litres of water an afternoon, or more if you're lively, sweat a lot or stay in a warm climate.

If you're frequently working up a sweat, is water enough? According to a 2004 look at on rehydration and healing after exercise , you want to consume a quantity of fluid extra than your sweat loss, together with eating enough replacement electrolytes.

Electrolytes encompass minerals like magnesium, potassium, calcium and sodium, and are determined in most ingredients. These minerals are vital to your frightened gadget, and they also get used up at some stage in muscle contraction. You can get sufficient electrolytes for muscle recovery via following healthful consuming behavior with lots of end result and vegetables. Having a tumbler of milk, coconut water or a fruit smoothie after your workout can help update electrolytes for your blood and resource healing.

Post Workout Snack

Grab a put up-exercise snack

After a workout, having a snack that consists of both carbohydrates and protein can help improve your muscle restoration time by way of providing the nutrients your muscle tissues needs to start repairing.

According to Sports Dietitians Australia, the body is simplest at replacing carbohydrates and selling muscle restore and growth within the first 60-90 minutes after you workout. Although this continues for any other 12-24 hours, maximizing your recovery in that first ninety-minute window is a awesome idea. The alternatives for quick, healthy snacks to top off your electricity stores are infinite — you could whip up a smoothie ahead of time, have a few fruit with yogurt, experience peanut butter or eggs on toast, or opt for a protein powder shake if you're in a rush and won't have the risk to consume for a while.

If you follow a plant-primarily based weight loss program, make sure you eat masses of excessive-protein foods at some stage in the day including nuts, tofu, quinoa and beans to present your muscle tissues the vitamins they need to restore.

Still hungry after dinner? A excessive-protein snack within the nighttime can fill the gap and useful resource muscle repair overnight.

Take a exercising supplement

While we are able to always inspire you to get your vitamins from whole ingredients, a few running shoes and athletes supplement with branch-chain amino acids (BCAAs).

A 2010 take a look at in the International Journal of Sports Nutrition and Exercise Metabolism showed that women who take BCAAs earlier than a exercising may additionally have much less submit-exercise pain and shorter muscle recuperation time.

For folks who already observe a wholesome weight loss program with sufficient protein, the use of supplements might not have a sizeable effect, as BCAAs are located in complete foods like eggs, animal protein, tofu, beans and dairy products.

Warm up earlier than resistance training

According to Mayo Clinic, taking the time to complete an powerful heat-up can also help to lessen muscle discomfort and the threat of damage.

A right heat-up is especially essential before hard workout routines and moves like deadlifts and pull-ups. Make certain your heat-up includes dynamic stretching to spark off the muscle tissues you're approximately to use, supporting to save you overstretching, stress or injury all through your exercising.

Make time to settle down

Alongside a warm-up, Mayo Clinic recommends cooling down after your workout to allow your coronary heart fee and blood stress to step by step get better.

Taking five-10 mins to walk on the treadmill can assist your body quiet down, particularly if you've just finished a tough workout or a HIIT session that actually got your coronary heart fee up!

Once your coronary heart rate has slowed, static stretching — in which you maintain a stretch role — can assist to enhance your variety of motion and save you you from feeling so tight the next day. Have hassle napping? A short stretching consultation before mattress may additionally help you to sleep better.

Foam Roll And Stretch

A 2019 meta-analysis of the outcomes of froth rolling on performance and recovery discovered that foam rolling before and after a exercise can also help improve performance.

Alongside dynamic stretching on your heat-up, foam rolling and stretching can enhance flexibility and help you get the most out of your education.

Tight hips are a commonplace trouble, so taking the time to stretch and foam roll can help lessen any pain, improve flexibility and assist your muscle healing.

Elevate your legs

It's usual to spend maximum of your time along with your legs down, whether or not it's sitting, status, lying down, strolling or going for walks.

According to the Cleveland Clinic, raising your legs or training the legs-up-the-wall yoga pose can assist with blood waft, swelling and the stream of physical fluids. Trying a few calming yoga poses can also help to improve flow.

Take a fab bath

Tough exercises can motive micro-tears in your muscle groups, which could bring about swelling, infection and soreness. This manner is ordinary, because the muscular tissues are adapting to the workload and turning into more potent.

If you're still sore one or days after your workout, taking a groovy tub or bathe can assist lessen irritation and support healing.

Some athletes additionally trust that cryotherapy — a treatment that involves exposing the frame to bloodless or close to-freezing temperatures — may help to appease muscle pain.

In a 2017 literature overview investigating the effect of complete-body cryotherapy (WBC) on healing after exercise, researchers observed WBC may additionally improve restoration from muscle damage, with enhancements in muscle ache and recuperation tending to come more consistently from multiple exposures.

If you have got a totally high degree of pain, soreness that lasts extra than five days, or need to attempt a brand new treatment, you should continually are searching for recommendation from a healthcare expert.

Rest For Muscle Recovery

Don't pass relaxation days

Alongside getting proper sleep, prioritizing your rest days can also help to hurry up the muscle repair procedure and depart you feeling refreshed and geared up to take in your next exercising.

With any worrying physical hobby, the American Council on Exercise (ACE) recommends scheduling at LEAST one day of whole rest (as opposed to an lively recuperation day) every 7-10 days to permit your body to get better and adapt. If you experience such as you want more relaxation - take it. Your body is aware of high-quality!

Keep transferring

Light movement in between your workouts can assist to keep the blood circulating for the duration of your body, bringing nutrients to restore the muscular tissues and supporting with the removal of metabolic waste.

A 2018 literature assessment posted in Frontiers in Physiology found that energetic restoration executed in the first few days of a hard exercise decreased the outcomes of not on time-onset muscle soreness (DOMS).

You might take the stairs, do a little stretching, or try to hit your every day step remember.

Wear compression tights

Research from 2019 at the effects of compression garments on recovery located massive nice results on overall performance, with researchers recommending athletes put on compression tights immediately after severe exercising primarily based on those outcomes.

Compression apparel might also help to reduce your belief of muscle discomfort and decrease infection and swelling.

The tightness of the material can help to promote blood waft via the deeper blood vessels in preference to the ones on the floor, which may resource with clearing waste and providing nutrients to the muscle fiber.

Reduce pressure

Did you understand that your emotional and intellectual wellness can affect your muscle healing?

When you're under strain, your body is targeted on its pressure reaction and has much less capacity to prioritize muscle recuperation.

A 2014 look at posted inside the Journal of Strength and Conditioning Research checked out whether continual mental strain affects muscle healing, perceived strength, fatigue, and soreness after strenuous resistance workout, over a 4-day duration.

The results showed that higher tiers of strain led to lower restoration and, conversely, lower degrees of stress have been related to advanced restoration.

Stress can also impact the whole thing from your sleep to ingesting patterns, hormones and preferred health. All of these things can impact your immune reaction, which is important for muscle restoration.

If you're underneath a number of pressure, strive the use of strategies like mindfulness and meditation, yoga, or make the time for interests you enjoy. Your pressure stages can be impacted by using a number of inner and outside factors, and if it's having a consistently negative impact on your each day lifestyles, reach out to a healthcare professional.

Follow the principle of innovative overload

Your training software shouldn't go away you feeling sore for days on cease after every workout. Ideally, any resistance schooling program will regularly boom the depth of each exercise, within your limits.

By applying the principle of innovative overload, you'll constantly project your body without pushing it beyond its present day threshold. This includes normal modifications for your exercise volume, depth, density and frequency.

Remember, simply because your muscle tissues don't hurt doesn't imply you didn't paintings hard or aren't making development!

Listen to your body

Sometimes at some point of or after a exercise, sure areas of your body would possibly sense tighter. These imbalances can occur as a end result of factors together with your way of life, behavior, anatomy and former injuries.

For example, in case you're proper or left-exceeded, one side will typically be stronger than the other and the weaker facet may experience tighter. You would possibly have tight shoulders from running at a pc all day, or a susceptible knee from an antique strolling injury!

Take a second after your workout to respire and cognizance on how your body feels — then you could tailor your quiet down primarily based on what your frame needs. You might spend a little extra time stretching one place that's tight and pay some interest to how it feels throughout your subsequent exercise.

Listening to your body additionally method understanding whilst to rest or reduce the intensity of your workouts, even in case your education software or fitness watch says to keep going!

Based on their findings, Sports Performance Bulletin says that at the same time as technology may be a useful manner to display overall performance and fatigue, you ought to by no means overlook the power of self-monitoring. Only YOU recognize how you genuinely experience - each in relation to fatigue, soreness and enthusiasm to your training. To keep away from burnout or overtraining, be aware about telltale symptoms like bad sleep, fatigue, decreased immunity or consistent achy muscle tissue.

Use these muscle healing thoughts to get better after your next exercising

Being sore isn't necessarily a sign of an amazing exercise, but, when you first begin a new workout application (or maybe a brand new exercising or schooling fashion!), muscle pain is very not unusual.

If you make a number of those changes for your ordinary and still find you're sore after each exercising or the pain lasts for extended intervals of time, recollect talking with a healthcare expert.

Chapter 9: The Banging Body

With exquisite strength, EVERYTHING we do is a great deal less difficult!

Life is a lot easier!

As time goes on, we're all going to end up weaker, and our muscle tissues are going to get smaller.

This loss begins in our thirties and will increase every decade after that.

This is NOT an inevitable component of growing old, though!

This is an unavoidable characteristic of acting less and less workout over time.

In this day and age, it is a whole lot simpler to do much less. It's a whole lot less difficult to be lazy!

When we don't HAVE to carry out matters that hold our muscle mass strong, we're going to grow weaker.

It's that easy!

Loss of muscle mass and power to gain the belongings you need and want to do, IS AVOIDABLE!

AND …. If you have got already realized you have misplaced energy and muscle….

It is REVERSIBLE as properly!

When you begin strength training (aka resistance training), in whatever shape - (as an example with weights, resistance bands or definitely performing body weight sports), and do it efficaciously, you WILL grow stronger, no matter your age!

a powerful older guy doing out with hand weights

That's correct any person over 60 can, at a minimal, keep their electricity and grow even stronger than a younger version of themselves.

And, with increasing electricity comes smooth mobility and getting greater out of life each day!

Furthermore, you'll also develop muscle, have more potent bones, reduce your hazard of falls, have much less discomfort, decorate your fitness, shed pounds, advantage confidence and look and feel better.

Sounds delicious, doesn't it?

Strength education is absolutely the maximum important form of exercising that all and sundry over 60 can do AND for my part, the maximum exciting!

powerful older woman with biceps

On the other hand, I know getting started with power training, especially with weights (or with resistance bands), may be a chunk tough or even intimidating.

If new to workout, it's difficult to know wherein to start, and plenty of questions may arise.

There also are numerous elements you need to take into consideration and execute to assure you acquire the consequences you desire and are not certainly losing it slow and putting yourself in danger.

With a touch know-how, though, energy training is VERY, VERY SIMPLE for everyone to begin into, and bring astonishing results. And that includes YOU!

In this e book, I'll educate you precisely the way to grow stronger, and explain simply how smooth it could be, even within the consolation of your own home.

By following this method, and being steady, it may not be lengthy until you are the more potent version of your self going approximately lifestyles without difficulty!

So without in addition ado, allow's turn out to be stronger!

THE BENEFITS OF STRENGTH TRAINING FOR SENIORS

Along with the advantages touched on in short earlier, there are numerous extra advantages of strength training, and this is why I accept as true with it's the maximum vital type of exercising that everyone over 60 can adopt.

Here are FIVE AMAZING BENEFITS of electricity schooling:

1. YOUNGER, STRONGER & MORE EFFICIENT MUSCLES

As time goes on and we come to be older, we lose strength, and we lose muscle tissues.

This procedure of our muscle mass being smaller and weaker with age is called sarcopenia.

There are several probably causes of sarcopenia. However, the good information is, inside the high-quality majority, sarcopenia is caused entirely through undertaking less physical workout at some point of the years.

Sarcopenia is NOT certainly an unavoidable indication of getting older.

It is an inherent indication of a loss of utilization.

When we adopt less physical exercising, our muscle cells get smaller and weaker.

By doing MORE bodily hobby, and training electricity workout routines, you may opposite the consequences of sarcopenia, successfully reversing the getting old method of your muscular tissues and enhancing their performance.

2. LOOK BETTER - LOSE WEIGHT & IMPROVE POSTURE

We ALL want to appearance better!

I'm sure it is fair to country that all people, both women and men, no matter age, seem better with a good amount of muscle on our frames.

We also look healthier with correct posture.

With regular electricity exercise (along side a healthy weight loss plan) you may broaden muscle groups, improve your posture (via resolving muscular imbalances), and decrease frame fats.

When you build muscle tissues and reduce fats, you get what is typically referred to as that "toned" appearance, which I recognize many of you analyzing this are pursuing.

Cardiovascular exercising (jogging, strolling, driving a motorbike, boxing, skipping, and so on) is the type of interest extensively seemed to be optimal for fats discount.

However, I'd pass as some distance as to argue that appropriate strength education can also do just as a lot, if now not extra, for weight reduction and weight manipulate as cardiovascular workout does.

Research reveals that electricity training results in decreases in stomach fat in each older men and women.

And next examine famous, finishing energy training resulted in just one-0.33 as lots fat boom over years compared to the ones no longer doing electricity education. Demonstrating the effect of electricity training on controlling weight. [10]

Now I am no longer advocating quitting training cardiovascular workout, specially in case you adore it.

There are blessings to conducting cardiovascular exercise for all and sundry over 60. However, in case you don't want to, you may become healthy, and robust and appearance your excellent with the aid of acting solely accurate power schooling.

three. IMPROVE PHYSICAL & MENTAL HEALTH & GET MORE, QUALITY SLEEP

Along with being more potent, developing muscle, dropping weight, and improving posture, power training can also decorate bodily and mental health.

For upgrades in our bodily fitness, power training may additionally lower the threat elements of metabolic syndrome, lowering blood stress [11, 12, 13] and lowering the risk of cardiovascular sickness.

It has tremendous consequences on levels of cholesterol and body fats percentage.

Strength training might also have a position in decreasing insulin resistance associated with ageing and preventing the improvement of diabetes.

Strength training may additionally make contributions to numerous intellectual fitness blessings.

After regular energy schooling, you may enjoy extra self assurance, vanity and feature extra energy. And, it is a effective method for minimizing strain and lowering tension, sadness, and weariness.

Moreover, if you need to hold your reminiscence in pinnacle form, power schooling may also enhance numerous elements of cognition, reminiscence, and reminiscence-associated sports in healthful older people.

And all of us realize the fitness benefits of getting a good night time's sleep. Resistance exercise may additionally growth sleep pleasant and amount.

4. DECREASE JOINT & OTHER PAIN. STRENGTHEN & AVOID BRITTLE BONES (HELP WITH ARTHRITIS & OSTEOPOROSIS) (HELP WITH ARTHRITIS & OSTEOPOROSIS)

Strength education facilitates save you and decrease discomfort. Studies have established a discount in ache in humans who have fibromyalgia, decrease back ache, and arthritis.

With painful joint illnesses together with arthritis, through strengthening the muscles, ligaments, and tendons around an afflicted joint, we might also minimize the pressure exerted on the joint, reducing ache sensations.

Strength exercising may also be powerful to prevent, and reversing osteoporosis. Studies have discovered will increase in bone mineral density, supporting to save you and support brittle bones.

Furthermore, stronger individuals are predisposed to have extra bone mineral density as compared to folks who are weaker.

5. PREVENT FALLS, DECREASE FALL RELATED INJURIES & IMPROVE BALANCE

Increased electricity and muscle tissues can also reduce one's risk of falls and pair with higher bone mineral density, significantly reducing the risk of fractures and other injuries related to falls.

Strength training has also been verified to be useful in improving balance and correcting age-related modifications in gait velocity (how speedy you stroll), stride length (the size of your doorstep), cadence (the pace of your stroll), and toe clearance (cleansing your feet off the ground with every step) [26]. All variables which are damaged, may also placed one in chance of falling.

As you can see, there are many, many lengthy-time period advantages of energy training and I desire by using now I've were given you over the line to begin strength training and start enhancing your lifestyles, and health.

Certainly, to experience all of the advantages and exercise power education well, you should do power schooling as it should be through following a few strategies which we are able to cross over within the next element.

Before we get into that, although, allow's tackle a few questions that you could have regarding strength education.

AM I TOO OLD TO LIFT WEIGHTS?

AGE IS NO BARRIER!

AGE IS JUST A NUMBER!

IT IS NOT THE END OF THE ROAD!

You are by no means too antique to perform some thing you want to do, and there are seniors all over the globe, displaying exactly this!

Take Irene O' shea who at 102 years old have become the arena's oldest skydiver.

Fauja Singh at 104 become strolling marathons.

Johanna Quaas at 92 - taking part in gymnastics.

Ernestine Shepherd is a Personal Trainer and maintains bodybuilding at 83 years antique.

You aren't too antique to carry out any form of weight schooling.

I have helped loads of people growth their strength and develop muscle from the age of 54 (or more youthful), all of the manner up to 104. 104 and flourishing!

You also are no longer too antique to accomplish some thing else you desire to do.

So, if you hold the idea that age is a purpose not to undertake whatever. Then chuck it out!

If a person tries to break your dreams with the "you're too vintage" excuse, toss them out too!

'Age' is by no means a cause to not accomplish some thing. Especially weights!

Whatever age you're, do some thing you want to do, and have a laugh doing it!

WON'T I HURT MYSELF IF I LIFT WEIGHTS?

If you enjoy this subject, you aren't by myself!

This is frequent anxiety encountered via people new to energy education, particularly in relation to lifting weights.

YES!

….. There IS a opportunity you may damage or injure yourself undertaking electricity workout routines!

And, our odds of harming oneself DOES grow as we grow old, and we DO growth our chance with the aid of training with weights.

However…. This concern is unjustified!

SHOULD WOMEN & MEN TRAIN DIFFERENTLY?

Again, No! To improve electricity for both men and women, the equal tips practice.

There is no want for gender-particular training to attain the energy profits you're pursuing.

If you desire to train alongside your associate, you may each adopt the identical exercise.

The primary distinction is that adult males, the bulk of the time, have higher energy degrees and large muscular mass. Meaning larger weights, or higher resistance could be essential to push oneself and advantage energy and muscle.

I AM A WOMAN & DON'T WANT TO GET 'BULKY'! WILL I GET BULKY IF I LIFT WEIGHTS?

So you've seen the photos of quite muscly women (usually competitive female bodybuilders) and have decided that lifting weights isn't for you.

No insult to these ladies who work pretty hard to obtain these physiques, however I can see, given loads of those photos, why lifting weights has been a no pass!

Although there is a completely high opportunity, you can awaken one morning, a bodybuilder huge after doing weights a few times, there's no want for this to throw you off doing weights.

I am in reality joking! The likelihood of this ever happening is close to none. I can assure you that you won't ever appear bulky!

Unless of direction you want to and are geared up to work very, very, very tough to gather it.

These muscled women have been doing weights for a long time (years and years), have tight diets, AND they're typically taking several supplements.

You aren't going to grow hefty like those girls! There is not any need to dread appearing power training.

And inside the improbable state of affairs, you do somehow, abruptly awaken with massive muscular tissues, applaud yourself! You have finished what others can not, specially at your age. Now to cast off these muscles which have nearly miraculously fashioned, sincerely go lighter at the weights (and consume much less) for a short time. You'll get back to now not being bulky right away.

As you can see, there may be no cause for this to prevent you from challenge power schooling.

older lady workout to tone her legs

Naturally, it takes A LOT of attempt for both ladies, AND guys, to seem muscular and expand 'cumbersome'.

What you may get with energy training, however, (and consuming an awesome weight-reduction plan) is greater muscle mass and much less fats over your muscle tissues, ensuing in that 'toned' appearance girls usually love.

HOW TO GET STRONGER OVER 60 (THE BASIC FORMULA) (THE BASIC FORMULA)

There IS a essential formula to expand stronger, but it's the equal for people of any age. Here it is

The Basic Strength Training Formula

1. Do exercising which includes resistance in a few manner, whether bodyweight physical activities or utilizing system (E.G. Weights or resistance bands) (E.G. Weights or resistance bands).

Make certain your muscle groups are being worked hard sufficient all through each workout (they develop weary - not exhausted), inside a sure set and repetition range (defined in a segment to comply with) (discussed in a section to follow).

2. Do this often every week, being careful to enhance the exercises while it gets too easy. Continue to assignment your self.

You can do that by growing the repetition variety (if doing bodyweight sporting events), doing a more tough variation of the exercise, lowering rest time, or growing the weight/resistance.

three. Support your strength training with right nutrition. Do not underestimate the significance of adequate vitamins for increasing energy and muscle tissues. To lose fats, getting your eating proper is up to 80-90% of the equation. If you're underneath-consuming or have a bad weight loss program, your strength will increase will be substantially constrained. (Nutrition for power can also be stated below).

Do these three steps, and also you WILL grow more potent.

It I.S. This is easy! You do not need to make it a great deal greater tough than this!

There are some extra nuances we're going to pass over to make sure you carry out each step perfectly, but that is the muse of it.

Stick to this system, and you can't pass incorrect!

Now, let's get into the nitty-gritty of power schooling, beginning with basic concepts to assure you get the maximum out of it and most significantly, do it properly.

STRENGTH TRAINING RULES TO STICK TO

So, now we know the fundamental, no-fail system important to grow more potent and gain muscle, and it's almost time we get into actual energy schooling.

However, before we delve right into it, we ought to pass over some fundamental power schooling policies, which whilst attended to, will preserve you secure throughout and can help you get the maximum out of your strength education.

RULE 1) SEE YOUR DOCTOR

I'm certain you know the drill....

As with any workout, there are hazards involved, and also you want to make certain you may exercise electricity schooling with out putting yourself at danger.

To supply yourself (and me) a piece of mind, consult your Doctor!

Get the all-clear before you start power schooling.

Also consulting a Health Professional, such as a Physiotherapist may be an awesome concept before you start power education for the primary time.

By doing this, you could discover ways to execute the sports with help and any regions of weak point may be dealt with first.

Once you have executed the subsequent, and you're all prepared to head, you could adequately begin your exercise.

RULE 2) ALWAYS DO A WARM-UP!

First and fundamental, earlier than commencing any activity, constantly and I imply ALWAYS whole a warm-up!

A warm-up is surprisingly important, especially with electricity sporting events or even greater so as we come to be older.

Properly warming up before operating out is important to prepare your frame for what follows.

Practicing at least a five-minute heat-up earlier than your real program, will not best lower your possibilities of being harm, or having different problems, but you furthermore mght put together your frame equipped for the energy workout routines that comply with.

The warm-up helps you with the aid of waking up your muscle tissues (and your self), lubricating your joints, and improving your variety of motion, enabling you to get greater out of the exercise.

To make things easier for you, I even have designed two heat-up exercises which might be easy to observe. Click underneath for the nice and cozy-ups.

STANDING WARM-UP ROUTINE

SEATED WARM-UP ROUTINE

STEP three) LEARN FIRST & USE GOOD EXERCISE TECHNIQUE

With each new workout, gaining knowledge of the right exercising technique first, before growing the burden, is a requirement!

If new to exercising, I propose beginning with bodyweight physical activities and reserve resistance bands and lifting weights for later, when you have obtained the technique and come to be a piece stronger.

This will assure no harm and assist you get the maximum out of the exercises, making them greater effective.

To ensure that you're as it should be completing the sports, reap a professional assessment, paintings with a training companion or execute the physical games in front of a reflect so you can see how it appears.

In this way, you may always monitor your exercise approach and regulate it if it starts offevolved to become worse.

Once you become snug along with your approach and sense that body weight isn't always pushing you enough longer, it is time to bring in some resistance bands or weights.

Only until you've got a super workout technique have to you consider bringing in greater weight/resistance to the sports.

Good workout approach goes to accomplish lots extra in acquiring the results you are searching out than the quantity of weight you are exercising with. So preserve affected person!

Once you begin making development, the idea is to enhance your energy gradually, and this may simplest be achieved safely, by means of step by step raising the load.

Your frame will respect you, you may stay harm-loose, and you may make notable progress through the years!

RULE 4) ALWAYS EASE INTO EXERCISE

When taking off strength training with weights (or bands) for the primary time, get started by using lifting lighter, and performing less than you are able to (fewer repetitions and units) (fewer repetitions and sets).

This gets your body acclimated to the exercise AND allow you to save you any pain or damage.

Soreness (DOMS) the following days after electricity exercising is perfectly normal and to be anticipated. But, you don't need to be in a whole global of affliction, which may occur in case you do too much!

Once you have mastered the strength exercises and were given your frame tailored to them, after some weeks, you may then start doing increasingly.

Another blunders I frequently see is people quitting appearing workout, or bodily interest, for an extended length (for specific motives) and finally, once they get lower back into the exercise, they attempt to begin back up where they left off. Avoid doing this!

You need to take a few steps lower back earlier than you get to in which you had been. This will reduce any risks of turning into harm and boost your results within the long term.

Always ease into motion, some thing it's far, in particular weights.

By doing this, you may keep away from any complications and be back to where you were very quickly!

RULE 5) DON'T LIFT TOO HEAVY

There may also come a factor when you are tempted to elevate bigger weights than you are able to.

You continuously need to be pushing yourself, however you do not ever need to be going past your limitations, leaving correct workout techniques at the back of and putting yourself in danger of injury.

Heavier weights with bad exercise technique accomplish nothing to develop your muscle tissues stronger and placed extra stress on other regions of your body.

Keep your weights within your capacity and SLOWLY improve the load over the years.

RULE 6) DON'T OVERDO IT, GIVE ADEQUATE REST & NEVER PUSH INTO PAIN

This one is quite much like what we mentioned above - the usage of a weight it truly is too heavy for you.

But pushing yourself over the boundaries would not always suggest using an excessive amount of weight; it may confer with over-workout additionally.

Getting stronger does now not require long, exhaustive exercising classes. This is senseless, putting big quantities of strain for your frame, and it'll work against you in getting the consequences you need.

You additionally want to present yourself rest between energy sessions. When we work our muscle mass with resistance, our muscle mass breaks down. Our body realizes it has to adapt to the brand new stressors it's far under and could start repairing and constructing stronger, larger muscular tissues which will cope with these physical activities once more.

Our body repairs itself via relaxation, sleep, and proper vitamins. So always supply your self good enough rest between energy education classes, specifically inside the beginning.

I recommend an afternoon in among every strength session and remembering to eat properly and continually get a good night's sleep.

Finally, bear in mind, sporting events have to NEVER cause you any ache. You may revel in a stretching feeling, fatigue, or that burning type of feeling of your muscle tissues being labored, and soreness the following day. But you ought to in no way sense pain.

This is why it is crucial to pay attention for your frame and prevent if it is causing you ache. You will understand when it would not feel proper!

Also forestall in case you enjoy some other unusual signs, along with chest pain, dizziness, or feeling faint.

RULE 7) STICK TO THE CORRECT SETS AND REP RANGES

To get the maximum out of your energy training, persist with an appropriate repetition and set levels.

We'll cover this in the following phase, however for now, know there is an quantity of workout we should stick to, so as to help us get more potent. And we'll get more potent quicker.

RULE 8) STAY CONSISTENT, ALWAYS BE CHALLENGING YOURSELF & PROGRESS THE EXERCISES

The ultimate tip to observe to guarantee you build your power is to be consistent.

Doing power education now and then isn't always going to boom your energy.

You should be performing electricity schooling, with out fail, each week. (We'll don't forget the frequency of exercises next).

Along with this consistency, as you develop more potent, you furthermore may want to be pushing your muscle mass by way of elevating the repetition levels (if performing bodyweight sporting events) or raising the quantity of weight (or the resistance of the bands), or you ought to exercise greater demanding activities.

If you don't hold to push your self, your power will in the end plateau out and also you won't turn out to be any more potent.

Always be pushing yourself! And remain steady!

Follow these guidelines to your strength education to exercise strength training effectively and to honestly acquire advantages.

With a clearer sense of what to perform, we now get to the electricity education elements that will first-rate develop your electricity – starting with how generally to exercising every week.

HOW MANY TIMES PER WEEK SHOULD SENIORS DO STRENGTH WORKOUTS?

a gymnasium diary, exercising footwear, and hand weights

To grow stronger and benefit muscle, you want to be exercise at the least twice every week and for more consequences purpose for 3 to four days per week.

Three days a week offers sooner or later in among to rest and recover from the exercises.

This is a first-rate technique to get your frame adjusted to this shape of the exercise with out pushing your self past the limit.

One electricity education according to week will no longer yield tremendous results and is perfect just for keeping power and muscle mass.

Consistency is the important thing to accomplishing outstanding effects.

If using bodyweight physical activities, or utilising extremely low weights, it's right to train every day. However, I suggest growing to larger weights/resistance to boost the efficacy of your electricity education, whilst those sporting events now not challenge you.

An example of a strength schooling exercise recurring, for beginners, can be:

2-days consistent with week, acting workouts on Monday and Thursday and finishing this for 4-6 weeks.

Once finished 4-6 weeks of education, you can pass to a few-days a week, training Monday, Wednesday, and Thursday. Allowing an afternoon in between exercises.

I advocate exercise each your decrease and higher frame every exercising.

HOW MANY REPETITIONS & SETS SHOULD SENIORS DO TO GET STRONGER?

Once you've determined how regularly you're going to do the workout routines each week, the subsequent step is knowing how in many instances to do each exercise throughout the exercising.

More especially, what number of repetitions, and units are required of every workout to get stronger?

For those now not acquainted with these standards, repetition (frequently called "reps") denotes how commonly you finish the exercise.

Performing a bicep curl, as an instance, for one repetition (rep) includes bringing your arm from a very straightened function to a totally bent function and returning to the begin position.

'10 reps' could mean performing ten complete actions of the exercising. So the use of the bicep curl example again, we take our arm from a totally straightened position to a totally bent function and then returned to the begin role and repeat this ten times.

A set way how often we do the ones precise range of repetitions.

Let's utilize "2 units of 10 repetitions" of the bicep curl as another instance. This manner we carry out 10 biceps curls at a time, take a little ruin and then do another ten biceps curls. Equaling two sets and 20 repetitions in general.

To grow stronger, there I.S. A specific repetition AND set variety you ought to stick with for maximum outcomes with energy.

Changing the repetitions and the units is going to goal various additives of health.

REPETITIONS

For Muscle Strength

If you find out you've got problems finishing actions like standing up, lifting goods, or ascending a few steps, your muscular power has actually reduced.

Lower repetitions, (1-6 repetitions) are the maximum beneficial for growing power. Heavier weights/resistance are essential for this repetition range.

I do now not recommend performing this low of repetitions, although, unless you have a excessive diploma of education OR you have a professional guiding you.

Keeping it simpler and more secure, I propose five-10 repetitions for seniors and modest weight.

This will enhance energy and additionally assist develop muscular mass greater effectively.

For Larger Muscles

If you discover your muscle groups have all started losing length, (i.E. Turning into smaller) that is referred to as muscular atrophy.

When muscle groups rises (length of the muscle), that is called muscular hypertrophy.

To enhance muscular mass, slight repetitions are gold standard, between 6-12 Repetitions.

I've determined repetitions higher than this, up to fifteen (every so often extra) also can work for constructing muscle.

For Muscular Endurance

If you find you can stand up pretty without problems, can raise items without problems, or even walk stairs without difficulty, it method your power is doing adequate. But, after a brief time of wearing an item, doing physical activities, or on foot round (either on the flat, upstairs or up hills) you start fatiguing, that could mean your muscular persistence has reduced.

Your muscular tissues have sufficient electricity to finish maximum of your movements however cannot hold this power/energy for an extended duration.

An instance of reduced muscular patience might be walking around a shopping center and feeling your legs fatigued and having to sit down down to rest.

To enhance muscular endurance, high repetitions of 15-20 repetitions and upwards will do this. And, lighter weights are essential. This repetition range also improves cardiovascular health and is beneficial for persistence sporting events inclusive of biking, strolling, or swimming.

Strength, hypertrophy, and staying power are all equally vital.

SETS

When it comes to the sets of each exercise to build energy and muscular tissues, even for endurance, the proof indicates a couple of sets are advanced to a single set.

Evidence additionally suggests that 2-five units are choicest for power, muscle tissues, and additionally patience.

So to construct energy, and hypertrophy and also paintings a few muscular endurance, I recommend 5-12 repetitions.

And 2-5 units.

To start, you may choose two units of 12, 3 units of 10, or four of eight.. All of those stages will help build strength. If getting began, start with much less. E.G. 2 sets of 8 and slowly increase the reps and units through the years. (and the weight).

If you keep to these tips, power teach often (at least days every week), and enhance the sporting activities by using continuing to push your self, you ARE going to grow stronger.

HOW HEAVY SHOULD MY WEIGHTS OR RESISTANCE BANDS BE?

There isn't any magic figure I can offer you for how heavy your weight or how thick your resistance band should be.

Everyone is different with numerous capabilities.

When beginning strength training, the most critical degree is getting to know the moves initially, the usage of frame weight or low weights.

As your strength begins to construct, you could steadily increase the load, making sure you keep away from any harm and have become the most out of your strength education program.

I do not propose lifting too heavy and training to complete failure. Ever! Training to fail approach lifting a weight where your muscular tissues are completely exhausted. This makes no sense! So make sure the load you pick out does not absolutely tire your muscle groups.

Instead, select a weight/resistance that isn't always too light that the exercise is a breeze, but heavy enough that your muscle tissues are very near being absolutely fatigued (getting close to failure, but no longer failure) via the remaining repetition of the ultimate set.

When exercise exclusive regions of your body, you're going to have one of a kind ranges of electricity. Leg exercises generally require heavier weight in comparison to arm sporting activities — a reason why it is a great idea to have a choice of weights and bands.

It's as much as you to determine how heavy your weights or resistance bands must be, and it receives less difficult as you come to be acquainted with the sporting activities (and the weights).

THE BEST RESISTANCE BANDS FOR SENIORS

resistance bands for seniors

Resistance bands bought off the internet will paintings pleasant to do most exercises with.

I advise going with ribbon type, and longer bands over shorter ones as this may can help you do greater physical activities and you may double them over or modify the scale your self.

If they may be too short, you're limited inside the workout routines you may undertake.

I recommend obtaining a few intensities from mild to heavy to allow for development.

If you outgrow the resistance bands, you could purchase thicker bands.

I am now inside the procedure of obtaining the exceptional resistance bands for seniors - This is in progress and to stay informed, ensure you're signed as much as the More Life Health e-mail list.

WHAT WEIGHTS DO YOU RECOMMEND? THE BEST WEIGHTS FOR SENIORS

type of bright hand weights

For weights, I additionally advise acquiring a modest set to keep money and permit for advancement as your strength grows.

For beginners, I suggest starting with 1-5kg (2-11lbs) weights. These are first-rate starting weights with a view to can help you research the moves, and that they offer an possibility for development.

When you outgrow these weights (a great problem to have), you can observe buying heavier weights.

Additionally, for the ones who've an awesome degree of power, you may need initially heavier weights.

If you maintain with the identical modest weights, your frame will not end up any more potent.

Progress the weight, via lifting heavier, and your body will adapt and grow more potent.

If you tour to your nearby department keep, you could absolutely select up a fixed of dumbbells.

However, to make things simpler, I actually have identified a few best beginning weight kits to help get you began.

Don't want to buy weights?

If you do not need to shop for weights or resistance bands, that is OK.

Although I do suggest ultimately getting device to gain continued boom, you may stick with the bodyweight physical games and enhance by way of putting in more reps as you advantage more potent over the years.

Or, you can virtually utilize materials you have round the house, together with water bottles or cans of food, so that it will work just best in the starting.

WHEN DO I PROGRESS WITH THE EXERCISES? - (USE HEAVIER WEIGHTS) (USE HEAVIER WEIGHTS)

As I've touched on during this publish earlier than when starting with weight schooling, the maximum vital level is that you grasp the proper exercising shape and make use of lightweight OR no weight in any respect. Keeping you secure and damage-loose.

Once you are finishing the workout properly, increase your weight. Use weights that your muscle groups are being worked on and move very near to exhaustion inside the repetition variety decided on (five-12) and set range (2-five). (2-five).

With consistency every week, your body will adapt to the exercising by means of developing stronger. When the weights or resistance bands become too low, it's far now time to raise them in slow increments. Choosing a bigger weight or resistance, that now accomplishes the aim of your muscle mass fatigue in the repetition and set range.

If at any second you undergo the repetition and set variety quick, using perfect workout form, and you're no longer close to to fatigued, it is time to raise larger weights/or utilize thicker resistance bands.

Other techniques to improve the sporting activities:

Do more repetitions (for bodyweight sporting activities)- Remember, but, in case you do too many repetitions, you'll shift into training muscular persistence in place of your power.

Do greater demanding sports - There are numerous approaches to adjust the exercises to cause them to harder. Take, for instance, a wall push-up vs a push-up on the ground.

Decrease your relaxation time among units. For instance, gently lessen by way of five seconds each week.

Or add in another batch after a while. If you begin with two units, continue to a few sets, and so on.

HOW LONG UNTIL I START SEEING RESULTS?

With accurate power schooling and sufficient nutritious consuming, you could expect to look and feel yourself developing stronger and subtle changes to your body pretty soon. From 1-2 weeks.

For novices, even as your frame is mastering the hobby, new neural (nerve) styles are put down among your brain and your muscular tissues.

Our muscle mass are made up of severa kinds of muscular fibers. Groups of those muscle fibers plus a motor neuron (nerve mobile) form what's called a motor unit.

Each motor unit has widespread portions of muscle fibers that if we don't utilize them, fall asleep. They lay inert until they're known as into motion again.

When you start strength training and preserve steady, your mind reacts to the workout by way of activating additional motor gadgets, waking up these previously latent muscle fibers, to coordinate the contraction of the muscle(s).

This growth in the previously sleepy, muscular fibers which might be now engaged to provide the electricity vital to raise the burden, explains why we may develop our energy as a substitute rapid.

When you adopt power workouts, your body is screaming "I cannot be susceptible longer, I need to be stronger to gain this", and your brain then wakes up your muscle mass to make it take place!

Increasing muscle tissues (hypertrophy), then again, will take a chunk longer

.

After continual strength schooling each week, for as much as 4-6 weeks or more, you will begin to sense your muscle tissue increasing. Like your biceps (see photograph) (see image).

Your muscle fibers are growing larger (hypertrophy), a good way to further improve your electricity.

If you've got accomplished strength education previously, although it turned into a long time ago, your frame will usually rebuild power and muscular tissues very rapidly (some thing called muscle memory) (some thing referred to as muscle memory).

NUTRITION: EATING TO GET YOU HEALTHY & STRONGhealthy food for seniors to promote fitness and well being

Eating healthily is crucial for fitness and properly-being, and is also important for growing muscle and enhancing strength. AND decreasing the waistline.

To develop more potent and expand muscle efficiently, we want to be consuming sufficient calories/strength from exquisite first-class protein, fat, and carbohydrate sources.

We also need to consume suitable micronutrients (vitamins and minerals) to guide our body's biological features and keep ourselves healthful.

When we're taking in too few calories, or ingesting specifically junk meals, we don't get hold of all our essential nutrients, ensuing in worse fitness and lack of muscle and electricity.

Nutrition is a large situation, hard to discuss in this educational. I could create an entire new guide on it. I'll save it for a later date, even though.

For now, optimize your food regimen with the aid of trying your excellent to avoid junk food, and begin receiving the proper range of energy from nutrient-rich ingredients.

There are specific nutrients you need to be eating enough stages of to resource enhance your energy (and health) likewise. That being protein, diet D, magnesium, and calcium, due to the fact low-degree intake of these nutrients, has been associated with decrease power, muscular mass, and physical overall performance in seniors.

Let's take a long examine these vitamins:

PROTEIN

steak with a vegetable salad

Protein is important for retaining muscular tissues, and energy, as one grows older, and it's fairly usual not to be receiving sufficient.

The Australian Dietary Guidelines suggest that 15-25% of our total calorie intake have to come from protein, with a each day consumption of the following:

The RDI of protein for women elderly 19–70 years is forty six grams in step with day.

The RDI of protein for adult males aged 19-70 years is 64 grams in line with day.

Women over 70 have to consume as a minimum 57g every day.

Men over 70 have to have above 81g each day.

However, new research have shown that protein consumption more than this can be important to retain muscular power and feature into a later age. [29, 30]

The European Society for Clinical Nutrition and Metabolism (ESPEN) makes the subsequent recommendations, primarily based on research accumulated:

1 - For healthful seniors - at the least 1.0 to at least one.2 g protein/kg body weight/day is usually recommended.

2- For seniors who are liable to malnutrition because they have acute or persistent disease, the food regimen should provide 1.2 to at least one.5 g protein/kg frame weight/day.

three - For seniors with severe sickness or damage - an even more consumption of one.2 to one.5 g protein/kg frame weight/day may be endorsed.

ESPEN additionally counseled regular workout and resistance education to keep fitness and muscular electricity and feature.

To discover extra about protein and get hold of suggestions on how to achieve more protein on your eating regimen, cross here.

VITAMIN D

We create diet D when our pores and skin is exposed to the sun. As we become older, we have a tendency to spend less time in the solar, especially in the winter months, making nutrition D shortages greater frequent.

beams of sunlight in a blue sky

Vitamin D is needed in older age for bone energy, muscular function, and keeping off falls.

Low nutrition D degrees are related with dwindled muscle tissue and negative athletic performance.

Aim to achieve 20 mins of direct sunshine each day, averting the warmest length of the day. This keeps your vitamin D ranges crowned up, supporting you stay healthy and powerful. Make cautious no longer to overuse it and burn your pores and skin.

MAGNESIUM

Magnesium is another mineral we need for maximum fitness.

seeds and nuts excessive in magnesium

Magnesium is essential for lots of our frame's basic activities, which include producing strength, neuron and muscle characteristic, production DNA, bone, and protein, and a wholesome heart and sturdy immune machine.

Decreased magnesium intakes were reported in seniors who've poorer muscular mass and power.

Furthermore, the intake of magnesium has been related to extended physical characteristic and electricity in seniors.

I'll be generating an article quickly to permit you to study more about magnesium and acquire guidelines on the way to acquire more magnesium in your food regimen. (preserve tuned for this).

CALCIUM

Calcium is wanted for strong bones and healthy teeth. It also plays a crucial element in different biological systems, inclusive of our neurological system and the appropriate functioning of our muscle mass.

milk and cheese high in calcium

Our traditional weight is made up of roughly two percent calcium. This calcium is largely positioned in our bones and tooth — the remainder is stored in our blood and tissues.

Poor calcium consumption has been related to osteoporosis, a low bone density disease maximum generally observed in put up-menopausal ladies.

Research has indicated that seniors with low calcium ranges, had a three-four times more hazard of sarcopenia and reduced gait pace, as compared to those with a higher calcium level

Strength education blended with an amazing weight-reduction plan, with appropriate energy, macronutrients (mainly protein), and micronutrients (which include diet D, magnesium, and calcium), is a solid technique to stopping sarcopenia and living a strong and healthful lifestyles.

Now, permit's study the best physical activities you need to use in your workout routines to get you stronger and make them extra effective

Several physical activities may be achieved to broaden power and muscular tissues. However, certain workouts are advanced to others and supply more utilitarian cost on your ordinary existence.

The sporting events that should be the center of any software encompass numerous joints and goal various muscle agencies. These workouts are referred to as compound physical activities. An instance of a complex exercising is the squat since it works the ankles, knees, and hip joints and numerous muscle agencies in your lower body.

Exercises that utilize just one joint and isolate positive muscle agencies are known as isolation sporting events. An example of an isolation workout is the bicep curl because the only joint moved at some point of the bicep curl is the elbow joint.

Isolation sporting activities nevertheless have their area in a training routine, but compound exercises might also goal these areas and are more effective and beneficial, leading to larger advantages.

Here are 5 of the greatest strengthening sports which I trust are important physical activities on the way to adopt to enhance electricity and bodily feature.

You may additionally perform those sports to your personal house as body weight exercises, or with resistance bands and/or dumbbells.

People who go to the health club may also be a part of a gymnasium software, and barbells may be applied with them.

If you have issues with the moves under, begin with sitting strengthening physical games.

1) THE SQUAT

There aren't too many other workouts that offer you the biggest bang in your dollar, like the squat.

The squat is an first rate exercise since it goals all the muscular tissues in the legs and the center.

The squat is a practical workout that trains the muscle mass essential to move about simply each day.

MUSCLES WORKED

Buttocks (glutes), thighs (quads), hips, calves, core, and back.

DIFFICULTY: Moderate

HOW TO:

Standing up tall with your feet shoulder-width apart.

Holding onto your chair with each hands.

Hinging on the hips and sitting again as in case you have been sitting on a chair.

As you sit down again, pass no further than 90 tiers, and as you stand lower back up.

Put same weight thru both legs.

Make sure your knees do not circulate above the line of your feet, and they aren't going inward during the workout.

Repeat for the given repetitions.

EASIER VARIATION: If you find the squat too tough, you may begin with a PARTIAL SQUAT or the SIT-TO-STAND.

PROGRESSING THE EXERCISE: This exercising can be made greater difficult by way of using no hands, resistance bands, dumbbells, or barbells.

2) THE DEADLIFT

The deadlift is similar to the squat inside the sense it makes use of all of the muscles in our lower frame (with greater hip involvement), however with the introduced of retaining onto the burden/resistance band. With the deadlift, we also educate greater of the returned

This workout is harder, so when you have difficulties with this, establish a goal, start with easy energy exercises and work your way up to it.

MUSCLES WORKED

Buttocks (glutes), thighs (quads), hips, calves, core, and returned.

DIFFICULTY: Harder

HOW TO:

Place your resistance band flat on the ground.

Sitting up tall closer to the the front of your chair.

Place your toes shoulder-width apart on the resistance band and face your feet barely outwards and preserve your knees in keeping with your ft.

Reach down and get keep of your resistance band and hold your upright posture along with your shoulders returned and down and your chest high.

Also, hold immediately fingers when protecting onto the resistance band, and maintain your shoulders back and down in proper posture while striking onto the resistance band.

Loosen or tighten the resistance band as needed to paintings your electricity.

From this posture, even as actually retaining onto the resistance, arise, precisely as inside the take a seat-to-stand workout now clinging onto the resistance band.

Ensure you straighten your legs and hips and squeeze your buttocks as you arrive at the height of the workout.

Now lightly sit down backtrack.

Keep equal weight thru both legs for the duration of the exercising and make sure your knees aren't shifting inward at some stage in the exercising.

Repeat for the given repetitions.

EASIER VARIATION: Lighter weight/resistance.

PROGRESSING THE EXERCISE: Using stronger resistance bands, utilizing no chair, the use of a barbell.

3) THE ROW

The row is every other splendid aggregate workout strengthening the muscular tissues of the higher again. Another first-rate useful exercising for everyday chores and enables a superb lot in improving posture.

This exercise is straightforward to finish, irrespective of your abilities. It may be done even as sitting or status and still makes use of the equal muscle tissue.

MUSCLES WORKED

Back, Arms, Shoulders & Core

DIFFICULTY: Easy to Moderate

HOW TO:

Stand up tall next to your chair and vicinity one hand on the chair

Now take a step lower back from the chair, with a slight bend inside the knees, hinge on the hips, bend ahead along with your back directly and area one arm by your aspect, maintaining it directly.

Now bending at the elbow, pull your arm up in the back of your back and return to the start role.

Squeeze your shoulder blades collectively while lifting your arm.

Repeat for the set repetitions and exchange fingers.

EASIER VARIATION: Lighter weight/resistance. Seated row.

PROGRESSING THE EXERCISE: Using heavier resistance bands or dumbbells, the usage of a barbell. If doing seated rows (a form of this workout), there may be a machine on the gyms where weight may be raised.

4) THE CHAIR PUSH-UP

In the preceding exercise, we exercised the muscle tissues worried inside the movement of pulling. In this subsequent exercise, we are going to deal with the muscle tissue involved while we execute a pushing action.

I even have picked the chair push-up for this due to its convenience of utilization in the home and being a chunk more difficult than a wall push-up.

A fashionable push-up is difficult for most, but if you may perform a everyday push-up, go for it! The equal goes with the changed push-up, with knees on the ground.

There are different sporting activities you can replacement for this depending in your capabilities, as an example, if the rush-up is simply too clean, you can do a bench press (or a press machine) at a health club.

Note: We have a tendency to make extra moves in the front of the body in our regular lives, which may lead to overworked muscular tissues at the the front, and weaker muscles on the rear of our body. This may lead to shoulder difficulties and bad posture. We should execute pull moves (for instance, exercise #3) greater often than push actions (this exercise) to balance the frame and beautify posture.

THE 10 BEST LEG STRENGTHENING EXERCISES FOR SENIORS

The legs are the most important part of the body to reinforce to guarantee you're moving about at your high-quality (and also lower the possibility of getting a fall) (and also decrease chances of having a fall).

The legs must be the major emphasis of any strength education for seniors.

Here are the five best leg strengthening sporting events for seniors to enhance leg energy.

Leg sports completed frequently will yield remarkable benefits. Many of your ordinary obligations will start feeling less complicated, and you will flow around with an awful lot extra consolation. You'll additionally feel steadier in your toes!

THE MOST SIMPLE STRENGTH WORKOUT FOR SENIORS TO GET AMAZING RESULTS

For the ones of you who lack the enthusiasm to get commenced and live with an exercise, I'm going to make it as simple as feasible to teach your complete body and acquire large improvements to your strength.

All I ask of you is that you undertake a simple routine with simply 3 movements and do them every 2d day.

If you stick to these physical activities, and always progress, through adding in extra repetitions, doing a extra difficult exercise, or adding in more weight. You will hold to get stronger and stronger.

Although different physical activities have their area too, those 3 physical games by myself will get your whole body more potent.

Strength schooling does not should be complex; preserve it easy!

These physical activities I actually have chosen paintings all the muscle groups to your legs, work your center, and the complete of the higher frame.

Chapter 10: The Benefit Of Balance Exercises

Balance sports enhance your ability to control and stabilize your body's position. This kind of workout is mainly essential for older adults. As you age, your ability to realize in which you are in space, known as proprioception, gets worse, which contributes to a decline in balance. These physical games also are vital for decreasing harm danger.

For instance, in case you sprain your ankle, you may be at threat for reinjury in case you do not retrain your balance. That's due to the fact whilst you sprain your ankle, the muscle groups around the joint stop contracting in a coordinated fashion, and this destabilizes the joint. If you do balance sports after the harm, it retrains the muscular tissues to settlement together, which higher stabilizes the joint all through actions and prevents re-injury.

A person desires to focus on improving their middle strength to improve balance, that may gain sports activities and different bodily activities.

How are you able to keep away from damage when doing stability sporting activities?

The main danger of doing stability physical activities is that you may fall. Make positive you have something near you that you can maintain on to in case you begin to fall. If you operate device which includes a balance board, you ought to make certain you are on a flat, strong, and non-skipper floor.

Start with an easy stability exercise, like moving your weight back and forth or status on one foot for some seconds, and progressively make your periods more hard — for example, by means of growing the time you spend on one foot, you need to begin on a strong surface and in a single role earlier than including any movements or stability exercise device.

How it really works

As with different styles of fitness, you may choose from a number stability physical games. However, all of them usually attention on improving someone's center and lower body power.

Before you start this exercise adventure

As with any exercising, you should communicate with a doctor about their overall fitness and health desires. The doctor can be able to guide physical activities to encompass or avoid based totally at the man or woman's ordinary health. You should communicate with a health practitioner about which physical games are great for you and take protection precautions while assignment any stability physical activities.

The American Heart Association (AHA)Trusted Source recommends that older adults interact in balance physical games on at least 3 days of the week. It also notes that someone may additionally desire to engage in exclusive exercises every day of the week.

If you are new to this kind of workout you must start with a simple habitual and regulate the sporting events as vital. As you construct extra self belief and electricity, you may increase the issue, period, and frequency in their sessions.

Balance exercises will help you enhance your stability, mobility, patience, and more, so this e-book discusses the distinctive styles of balance sporting events and their advantages for older humans.

Chapter 11: The Balance Exercises

Seated Exercises

Ankle and Wrist Rolls

Many seniors war with poor stream thru the extremities, which can make contributions to obstacles with balance and mobility, "waking up" the fingers and toes via a chain of lower-intensity movements is very necessary before diving into extra rigorous exercises.

How To Perform This Exercise:

. Sit tall on a take a look at chair, so your lower back is instantly and isn't always leaning in opposition to the chair lower back.

Flex your arms, starting and closing your fists several times before making fists and rolling your wrists 10 times in each route.

Perform the equal physical games together with your feet. First, flex and factor every foot independently as you simultaneously curl and straighten your feet.

One at a time, roll every ankle to the outside 10 instances, then separately, roll every ankle to the inside 10 instances.

Single-Leg Calf Raises

Calf increases can growth power and mobility via the decrease leg, and may be finished sitting down.

How To Perform This Exercise:

Sitting tall in a chair with ft planted flat on the ground approximately hip distance aside, engage your core and appearance straight ahead.

Start with the right foot and raise your heel from the floor as excessive as you may, seeking to improve as high as you can to your ft, attractive the calf as you perform the workout. Lower the heel returned to the ground and repeat to finish a fixed of 10 repetitions.

Repeat the motion with the left leg.

Perform three sets of 10 reps in keeping with leg.

After acting the preliminary units, add two more sets of 10 repetitions, this time lifting both heels simultaneously. At the quit of the last set, preserve the heels lifted from the ground for 20 seconds.

Sit-and-Stands

For older adults who can also struggle to stand up from low chairs or gentle couches. Sit-and-stands—a precursor to squats can assist seniors advantage or keep the potential to get inside and out of chairs independently, improving leg strength, practical stability, and manipulate.

How To Perform This Exercise:

Start seated in a examine chair, ft planted on the floor about hip distance aside.

Using as little help from fingers or arms as possible, have interaction your core, and tip ahead from the hips.

Press your weight via all 4 corners of your feet and push yourself to stand, extending your knees and hips fully.

Reverse the motion, pressing your hips returned and bending your knees to carefully lower yourself to the seated position.

Seated Hip Marches

For individuals who need to enhance flexibility and mobility thru the hips, or who want a modified choice for appearing cardiovascular exercise, seated hip marches are an awesome desire.

How To Perform This Exercise:

Sit tall on a study chair, your toes flat at the ground, hip distance apart.

Grasp the edges or armrests of the chair with each hands and interact your abdominal muscle tissues to assist keep your torso tall.

Lift your right leg together with your knee bent as high as you readily can, as though doing a excessive-knee march.

Lower your right foot to the floor with manage.

Repeat to the alternative facet.

Perform at least 20 alternating marches in succession. Take a wreck, then repeat two to a few extra times.

This workout may be persevered for a greater cardiovascular impact, or it can be integrated into a heat-as much as assist increase the heart fee and get the blood flowing before appearing extra energy-centered movements.

Heel Slides

Heel slides are a type of modified hamstring curl designed to help make stronger the massive muscle groups spanning the lower back of the thigh among the glutes and the knees. Because core engagement is needed, the workout can also expand stomach energy.

How To Perform This Exercise:

Sit tall in a robust chair, with knees bent and feet flat on the ground about a hip distance apart.

Extend the right leg and flex the right foot, so the heel remains in touch with the ground, but the feet are pointing up in the direction of the ceiling.

Engage your glutes and hamstrings, the usage of these muscle groups to tug your proper heel back towards the chair while it remains in touch with the floor.

Reverse the movement and slide your heel away from you, extending your proper knee. Perform 10 to twelve repetitions on one side earlier than switching legs.

Complete to 3 units in keeping with leg.

While this workout can be done without any special device, you may need to apply a paper plate or a small towel to make it less complicated for the heel to slide across the ground.

Seated Shoulder Press

It is essential to contain electricity-training sporting events that easily translate to useful every day activities.

Overhead arm raises with or without weights are a notable way to exercise placing objects away on cabinets or in overhead boxes.

In addition to developing electricity, this type of overhead lifting movement takes the shoulders through a complete variety of movement which helps maintain flexibility via the shoulders.

Use light-weight dumbbells, water bottles, canned goods, or resistance bands to carry out this workout. If you're using a resistance band, select an extended, flat band and steady it in vicinity via sitting on top of the center of the band earlier than greedy each stop to perform the exercise.

How To Perform This Exercise:

Sit tall in a examine chair, your toes flat on the floor approximately shoulder distance apart.

Hold a mild dumbbell or the cease of a resistance band in every hand at your shoulders, your elbows bent and your arms facing far from you.

Press your arms straight up overhead, extending your elbows.

Carefully decrease your palms again to the beginning role.

Complete two to three sets of 10 to 12 repetitions.

Modified Leg Lifts

A chair-based modified leg raise let you enhance core strength. While it's nice to apply a robust chair with armrests for this flow, you may also perform the exercise at the same time as gripping the rims of the chair beside your hips.

How To Perform This Exercise:

Sit tall in a chair, your middle engaged, your toes collectively and flat on the floor. Roll your shoulders returned to keep best posture.

Hold the chair's armrests or grip the chair's seat. Keeping your feet and knees together, lift both legs as excessive as you can (with knees bent) as you exhale.

Hold for 5 seconds, then decrease your ft returned to the floor.

Perform 10 to 12 repetitions and complete a complete of three to 5 units.

Band Pull-Apart

Many seniors have rounded backs, so it is crucial to paintings the posterior chain to preserve the chest open and the lower back strong. The band pull-apart workout enables correct posture.

How To Perform This Exercise:

Hold a mini resistance band in front of you with both of your hands

Draw your elbows out extensive and pull the band.

As you pull the band, squeeze your shoulder blades collectively to interact your lats and rhomboid muscular tissues.

Slowly go back your arms to the starting function.

Standing Exercises

Sit-to-Stand

Standing up from a chair or toilet is a primary factor for seniors being able to stay at home independently. Otherwise, a few may additionally want to hire a complete-time resident assistant or go to an assisted living community. It's additionally essential to recollect that spending too much time sitting can be potentially risky on your fitness. This exercise for seniors strengthens the muscle tissues on your upper legs.

How To Perform This Exercise:

Stand in the front of a chair along with your feet aside and your palms immediately out in front of your shoulders.

Holding your arms out will help you stay balanced as you whole repetitions.

Bend your knees and push your hips down in the direction of the bottom of the chair.

After a slight pause, press your body upward and rise up to finish the rep.

Two to three units of 10 reps a day are encouraged.

Tandem Stance

The tandem stance is in the main used as a way to check your stability. But, it is also an amazing workout for seniors to carry out each day. For extra methods to help improve your stability, take a look at out the high-quality balance exercises to improve your balance.

How To Perform This Exercises:

Stand together with your ft collectively and your hands instantly out in your facets.

Put one foot in the front of the other in a instantly line and maintain this function for 30 seconds.

Switch the placement of your toes and repeat.

Holding your fingers out on your aspects will help you stay balanced.

Farmer's Walk

This status workout for seniors works out your higher body and promotes core electricity. Perfecting complements your ability to do any day by day workout or pastime which you want to do.

How To Perform This Exercise:

Stand tall together with your feet hip-width apart and a weight in every hand down by way of your facets.

From right here, slowly walk ahead for 30 seconds then repeat within the opposite route.

Flamingo Stand

This entails standing on one foot for a brief duration.

It entails this series of moves.

How To Perform This Exercise:

Stand up immediately, near a wall, chair, or every other robust object.

Shift the weight onto the right foot and raise the left foot off the floor, bending the knee to bring the heel close to the buttock.

Make positive your center isn't leaning closer to one aspect of your frame.

If important, vicinity the right hand at the wall or chair for assist.

To make the exercising more challenging, reach for the left foot with the left hand.

Hold the foot for up to fifteen seconds.

Place the left foot lower back at the ground and repeat with the proper foot.

Tightrope Walk

How To Perform This Exercise:

Place a chunk of string or ribbon on the floor.

Hold the hands out to the perimeters.

Walk alongside the string, setting the feet at once on it.

Walk as a minimum 15 steps.

Repeat the workout as favored.

Walking Exercises

Walking offers your complete device a boost and can be a key part of a healthful and unbiased senior way of life.

For first-rate outcomes, be affordable and practical whilst beginning your on foot routine. The concept is to provide yourself the advantages of exercise at the same time as mastering your limits and mastering your very own frame.

Start Smart

The secret to a a success walking software is deciding on a practical plan and sticking to it. Don't be overly bold. The massive blessings of on foot come over the years. Tailor a while and electricity output to the appropriate stage in your age and health popularity. Guidelines from the Centers for Disease Control and Prevention suggest that older Americans interact in slight to mild cardio workout for at the least 2.5 hours in step with week. Spread out over seven days which interprets into approximately 20 minutes an afternoon. This guideline isn't a tough and speedy rule but, pick out what is proper for you and build your walking software at your personal tempo.

Warming up

Before launching a energetic strolling application make certain that you heat up your muscle groups and do a balance take a look at.

Start slowly. Stand up immediately and lift your fingers above your head. If you are feeling consistent, rotate your hands in a windmill movement. This receives your blood going and loosens up your arm and shoulder muscle tissues. If you feel unsteady, stand behind a chair and maintain onto it with one hand. Practice lifting one foot and then the opposite. This slight stability exercising can help prepare you for your strolling software.

Setting the Pace

Before you start, understand in which you are going. Choose a direction that you're acquainted with and begin sluggish. A flat and large surface with out too many hills is quality for beginners. Use your complete body, which include your palms, as you stroll. Swing your hands backward and forward with an clean movement -- however do not overdo it -- it should not harm. When you include arm movement into a strolling habitual you work your complete torso and maximize aerobic benefits. Set a realistic pace to begin and deliver yourself at least 5 to ten minutes at that pace before you begin to push yourself.

Path to Power Walking

A everyday and constant walking routine can be a constructing block to a extra vigorous cardio and strength schooling gadget. When you've gotten to realize yourself and your potential you could begin which include some additional features into your strolling application. Strength schooling is an clean one to feature Start small with a 1 or 2-pound weight in every hand. Weights have to no longer experience too heavy. Try lifting each weight among 8 and 10 times. If this isn't always tough, then the burden is proper for you. If you cannot raise and repeat eight instances, then the burden is just too heavy. Once you get it proper, walk your usual path with your hand weights for a incredible full-body exercise

Core Exercises

Core physical games are those sporting activities that target the stomach muscle tissue.

These muscular tissues, positioned at some point of a lot of your trunk, are the important thing to supporting your decrease returned and supporting you stand, get out of a chair, bend, elevate, and hold your balance. So everyday upkeep and track-united statesof the center muscle tissues are vital.

Your middle muscle tissues offer balance for the transferring components above and below them — the mid-returned, or thoracic, the backbone that enables you twist and flip, and the hips that flow you up, down, back, or forward.

Which muscle tissue make up the center?

Generally speaking, the core starts offevolved on the lower rib cage and extends to the buttocks.

Core muscle tissue in the stomach consist of the lengthy rectus abdominis muscle tissue within the the front; the external and inner obliques on the edges; and a extensive, flat girdle in the front called the transversus abdominis.

If you haven't worked on your middle in a long term, I suggest you start slowly, focusing on the first-rate of the workout and gradually growing the wide variety of instances you can do it.

Unlike a few muscle agencies that should simplest be labored out each other day, center muscle groups may be strengthened daily. The core should constantly be working.

Remember to do a warm-up earlier than strengthening. March in place for a couple of minutes and pass your arms around to get the blood flowing.

After strengthening, stretch your muscle groups, in particular the hip flexors within the front of your pelvis and the hamstrings inside the returned of the thighs.

The quality core exercises

A much better method to strengthening your core is operating for several middle muscle companies on the same time, just the manner you'll clearly in case you have been lifting some thing or mountaineering.

Bridges

Anyone can do a bridge. You begin in a recumbent position for your returned and then raise and hold your buttocks off the floor. It's effective due to the fact you create stress from the rib cage to the pelvis and from the belly button around to the back. The entire vicinity turns into solid, and it creates a contraction of all of the muscle groups, like a corset.

How To Perform This Exercise:

Lie to your again along with your knees bent and ft flat on the ground, hip-width apart.

Place your arms at your sides. Tighten your buttocks, then carry your hips off the ground until they shape a straight line together with your hips and shoulders. Hold.

Return to the starting role. Repeat 10 times.

Planks

Planks create contractions of the center, arm, and shoulder muscle mass as you live in a push-up role. The secret is staying as stiff as you could, like a timber plank.

How To Perform This Exercise:

Start to your hands and knees. Tighten your belly muscle tissues and decrease your higher frame onto your forearms, aligning your shoulders at once over your elbows and keeping your ft within the air at the back of you.

Keep your returned directly, making your frame as much like a "plank" as viable.

Hold the placement and return to the starting role. Repeat 10 times

www.ingramcontent.com/pod-product-compliance
Lightning Source LLC
Chambersburg PA
CBHW060500030426
42337CB00015B/1665